PANDEMICS
A HISTORY

A Golden Meteorite Press Book.
Printed in Canada.

© Copyright 2020, Austin Mardon, Alex Elvidge, Mya Colwell, Sriraam Sivachandran, Michael Tang, Catherine Mardon

Golden Meteorite Press, Edmonton.
All rights reserved for Pandemics: A History©.
No part of this publication may be reproduced, stored in any retrieval system, or transmitted in any form or by any means, electronic, mechanical, photocopying, recording, microfilm reproduction and copying, or, otherwise, without the prior express written permission of Golden Meteorite Press:

First Printing: 2020

Design and layout by Jacob Rose

Telephone: 587-783-0059
Email: aamardon@yahoo.ca
Website: goldenmeteoritepress.com

Additional copies can be ordered from:
Suite 103 11919-82 Street NW
Edmonton AB
T5B 2W4
CANADA

ISBN 978-1-77369-174-9

We acknowledge the support of Canada Service Corps, TakingITGlobal, and the Government of Canada in promotional materials associated with the Project.

Thank you

PANDEMICS
A HISTORY

*Austin Mardon, Alex Elvidge, Mya Colwell,
Sriraam Sivachandran, Michael Tang,
& Catherine Mardon*

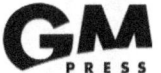

Table of Contents

Introduction **13**
    Terminology 13
    All Living Organisms Are Just Trying to Survive 14
    Disease Historiography 17
    What Makes a Disease Famous? 18
    Notable Mentions 20

Chapter 1: Antonine Plague (165-180) **25**
    Galen and Smallpox 27
    Spread and Symptoms 28
    Impact 30

Chapter 2: The Plague of Justinian (541-549) **33**
    The Journey of Yersinia pestis 34
    The Humble Flea and the Well-Travelled Rat 36
    Symptoms 39
    Impact 40

Chapter 3: The Black Death (1346-1353) **43**
    The Crisis of the Late Middle Ages 43
    The Second Journey of Yersinia pestis 45
    Symptoms 47
    Impact 48
    What Caused It? 49

Chapter 4: Smallpox **52**
    Introduction 52
    Symptoms 52
    The Spread of Smallpox 54
    From Magic Lozenges to Vaccination 56
    Anti-vaccination 58
    Eradication 59
    Conclusion 60

Chapter 5: 17th Century Great Plagues ... 61
Introduction ... 61
Symptoms ... 62
The Plague in 17th century Europe ... 63
The Plague enters London ... 64
Measures taken to slow the spread ... 65
Public Reception ... 67
Treatment and Precautions ... 68
Conclusion ... 69

Chapter 6: Cholera (1817-1923) ... 70
Cholera: A brief overview ... 70
Symptoms ... 71
The First Cholera Pandemic (1817-c.1826) ... 71
The Second Cholera Pandemic (1829-1852) ... 72
The Third Pandemic (1852-1862) ... 74
The Fourth Cholera Pandemic (1863-1879) ... 75
The Fifth Cholera Pandemic (1881-1896) ... 77
The Sixth Cholera Pandemic (1899-c.1923) ... 77
Treatment ... 78
Conclusion ... 79

Chapter 7: The Third Plague (1855) ... 80
Symptoms ... 81
The Spread ... 82
Germ Theory ... 83
Rats and the Plague ... 84
Preventative Measures ... 85
Conclusion ... 87

Chapter 8: Spanish Flu (1918 – 1919) ... 89
Background ... 89
The First Wave ... 91
The Second Wave ... 92
The Third Wave ... 93
Impact ... 94
Conclusion ... 95

Chapter 9: Asian Flu (1957 – 1958) 97
Impact and Spread. 97
Symptoms 99
Response 100

Chapter 10: Swine Flu (2009 – 2010) 104
Background. 104
Symptoms 106
Treatment 108
Response 109

Chapter 11: Ebola Virus (2014 – 2016) 111
How did it start?. 112
Contraction and Transmission 114
Symptoms 115
Treatment 116

Chapter 12: COVID-19 118
An overview of COVID-19 118
Symptoms 119
International response 119
The role of the WHO during the pandemic 121
Infection control 123
Potential treatments and vaccines for COVID-19. 125

Chapter 13: Future Pandemics 126
Preventing and fighting pandemics in the future 126
The largest source of human diseases: Wildlife 126
Investing in research and databases 127
Improving healthcare systems 129
Improving infrastructure and urban design. 130
Taking advantage of technology 132

Chapter 14: The Evolution of Pandemics 134
The evolution of pandemics. 134
Recurring patterns in most pandemics 134

Agriculture, the wildlife trade and habitat exploitation 136
Trade, travel and exploration 137
Warfare and conquest 138
Developments in medicine, public health 139
Developments in research, technology and infrastructure. 140

Conclusion 143
The impact of pandemics 143
Potential next steps 145
A final message 149

Works Cited 151

Author Bios:

Alex Elvidge has a Master's in Classics from Queen's University and resides in Ottawa, Ontario.

Mya Colwell is pursuing a Bachelor of Communication Studies at MacEwan University and resides in Edmonton, Alberta.

Sriraam Sivachandran is pursuing a Bachelor of Science at McMaster University and resides in Markham, Ontario.

Michael Tang is pursuing a Bachelor of Health Sciences degree at Queen's University and resides in Toronto, Ontario.

World Diseases Deathtoll:

Disease	Deaths
Antonine Plague (165-180 AD)	●●●●●
Plague of Justinian (541-532 AD)	●●
The Black Death (1346-1353 AD)	●●
The Great Plague of London (1665-1666)	●
The Third Plague (1855)	●●●●●
Smallpox (20th century)	(500 dots)
Spanish Flu (1918-1919)	●●
Asian Flu (1857-1958)	●●
Swine Flu (In 2009)	●
Ebola virus (2014-2016)	●
Cholera (Every Year Today)	●
COVID-19	●

● = 1,000,000 Deaths

Highest estimations shown.

Introduction

Alex Elvidge

If there has been one unequivocal constant throughout the history of human life, it's disease. Humanity has been struggling with the effects of disease since the dawn of civilization. As farming developed with the agricultural revolution and communities expanded from small isolated groups to sprawling metropoleis, the wider and more rapid spread of disease has been a natural consequence faced by every accessible nation and individual worldwide.

Terminology

Not all infectious disease terminology is created equal, though often mistakenly this terminology is used interchangeably. The difference between an epidemic and a pandemic, for instance, is a matter of scope – while "epidemic" is used to categorize a disease that affects a large number of people within a community, population, or region, "pandemic" is used when an epidemic spreads to a wider geographical scale, affecting multiple countries or continents and a large portion of the global population.[1] On March 11th, 2020, the World Health Organization officially changed its designation of COVID-19, the illness caused by coronavirus, from an epidemic to a pandemic. There is no quantitative agreement on how widespread a disease must be in

---

1   Both of these terms have ancient Greek origins, with "epidemic" being derived from the words ἐπί ("on" or "upon") and δημός ("the people" or "the country") meaning "upon the people", and "pandemic" being derived from the words πᾶν ("all, every") and δημός, meaning "all the people".

order to become classified as an epidemic or how widespread an epidemic must grow in order to become a pandemic. Therefore, the distinction between such terminology is regularly blurred because the definition of each term is fluid, changing as diseases become more or less prevalent over time, and as flare-ups occur and diseases begin to spread.

In light of the present global pandemic, many people are currently engaging in regular conversations about infectious diseases that they might not normally have. In such conversations, and in the following book, you might come across terms such as "endemic" or "outbreak" – these refer to whether a disease is regularly found among a particular group of people or within a certain area. Endemics are used to refer to diseases that are a constant presence in a particular location – for instance, Malaria is endemic to parts of Africa. However, an outbreak is what occurs when a disease appears in an area where it is not endemic. A recent example comes from 2019 – dengue fever is endemic to certain regions of Africa, Central and South America, and the Caribbean, as mosquitoes in these areas carry the disease and transmit it from person to person. However, last year there was an outbreak of dengue fever in Hawaii, where the disease is not endemic. It is believed a person from one of the endemic regions infected with dengue fever visited Hawaii, was bitten by a mosquito there, and that mosquito began spreading the disease to individuals in Hawaii, thus creating an outbreak.

All Living Organisms Are Just Trying to Survive

One's susceptibility to a particular infection or virus varies from community to community and even from person to person.

Such differences are sometimes hereditary, but typically these differences are the result of past exposure to the disease in question. Adjustments of human defenses against disease occur all the time, not only within individual bodies but among entire populations. However, just as humans undergo continuous alteration to adapt their defenses to infectious disease, so too do infectious organisms that provoke disease adapt and adjust to their environment. Parasites need a host to survive, and they are just as concerned with their own survival as we are with ours. This is not always a bad thing – yes, it is disheartening that a virus can often learn to maneuver around our defenses just as quickly as we can build them. But sometimes, a virus will adapt itself to be less deadly so that it can survive long enough to spread to another host – if a virus kills off its host too quickly before it can spread, the virus dies too. All living organisms are just trying to survive.

    An example of an infection that burned through its host population so quickly and with such force that the impact, though high in mortality, was relatively short-lived, is also one of the earliest known well-documented epidemics in history, occurring over 2,500 years ago. In 430-426/7 BC, during the Peloponnesian War between Athens and Sparta, a disease which many now believe to have been a form of typhoid fever struck the Mediterranean. While the Peloponnese escaped the effects of the epidemic known as the Athenian Plague nearly unscathed, Athens was hit harder than elsewhere in the Classical Greek world because the city was under siege and crowded with people. Over the course of four years, the plague killed a quarter of the Athenian troops and an additional quarter of the general Athenian population. Thucydides' description of the plague in his *History of the Peloponnesian War* is known as one of the great passages of Greek literature.[2] Though this epidemic greatly

---

2   Thuc. 2.48-54.

weakened Athenian dominance over the surrounding Greek poleis and made a major contribution to Athens' ultimate loss of the Peloponnesian War, the sheer virulence of the disease prevented its spread to the wider Mediterranean and the Near East – it killed off its host at a faster rate than it could spread. Thucydides writes, "Appalling too was the rapidity with which men caught the infection; dying like sheep if they attended on one another, the sufferers died in their solitude, so that many houses were empty because there had been no one left to take care of the sick; or if they ventured they perished, especially those who aspired to heroism."[3]

Thucydides, known today as one of the greatest and most prolific ancient historians, described in detail the effects of the Athenian Plague, both on the individual and in regard to the devastation of the city. He wrote that the dead lay right where they had died, piled one on top of the other, "while others hardly alive wallowed in the streets and crawled about every fountain craving for water," and temples were filled with the corpses of those who had died in them. He also described how the plague affected the moral attitudes of the Athenian citizen – individuals were reduced to their basest urges and began openly committing crimes, either because the city was in such a state of disarray that they knew they could get away with it, or because the hopelessness wrought by the devastating surrounding them made them careless of the consequences. According to Thucydides, "they resolved to enjoy themselves while they could, and to think only of pleasure." The effects of the plague were of a magnitude "nowhere remembered".[4]

---

[3] Thuc. 2.51.

[4] Thuc. 2.52-53.

Disease Historiography

The reader may notice that more than half of the chosen pandemics in this book are from the last 200 years. This is not because plagues have become more frequent since the 19th century. In fact, infectious diseases were undoubtedly a very important factor in the high death rate of the ancient world in all periods. Great epidemics and pandemics were nothing new. However, the farther we progress in history, the more detailed and accurate our accounts of major diseases become. Documentation of more recent pandemics is considerably more complete, in large part because of greater reliability of statistics, which allows the proper record-keeping of population size, mortality rate, total death toll, etc.

Often, especially on the subject of antiquity, the fame of certain events owes itself in large part to either accident or exaggeration. The written accounts and physical evidence that remains extant for us today survives in large part by accident. Just because we have a relatively detailed account of a particular plague from the ancient world does not necessarily indicate that this was the only plague in hundreds of years, or even that it was a particularly bad plague of the time, so devastating that people felt compelled to document its effects. It could simply mean that the accounts of other plagues and diseases that cropped up throughout the centuries have since been lost, destroyed by time or by war, or discarded by disinterested hands. As it is, the Antonine Plague from the 2nd century AD often follows after the Athenian Plague of the 5th century BC in historical accounts, with the two plagues mentioned right after the other as if no other major diseases had popped up in the 600-year gap between them. There is a reason for this: the interests of past historians and biographers, on whom we largely depend for this information, tend to lie in major wars, events, and historical figures. Not nearly as much would have been made of these two particular plagues if they had not been connected with such significant occurrences and individuals. The Athenian Plague ticks 4 of these boxes: 1) it occurred at a crucial point in the Peloponnesian Wars, and 2) resulted in the famous Funeral Oration by 3) Pericles, a prominent Athenian general who, not to mention, actually died from the plague, and 4) was subsequently documented by the widely-read historian Thucydides. Thus, the Athenian Plague survives the destruction of time and history. The Antonine Plague, meanwhile, was 1) connected to major battles in which emperors took command, and 2) directly affected the city of Rome itself. Not to mention, 3) Galen himself described the pandemic, and thus this plague too survives history. From the perspective of historian J. F. Gilliam, if Galen had lived under any other emperor than Marcus Aurelius – perhaps Augustus, or Nero, or Titus, or Hadrian – and had described one of the many plagues which occurred in their own reigns, modern history would likely remember another great plague, and the one under Marcus Aurelius would have been lost to history.[5]

What Makes a Disease Famous?

The historical plagues discussed in this book were chosen because they can each be classified as major pandemics that resulted in high death tolls and great social disruptions over large areas of the world. However, the historical and humanitarian significance of a pandemic does not derive solely from its mortality rate. Particularly when discussing events from antiquity, proper estimates of death tolls can be unreliable or exaggerated.

---

5   Gilliam 1961: 248.

Some plagues have impacted communities and cultures more severely than their death tolls might suggest. Some pandemics are particularly worth exploring because they ignited a response that significantly altered or advanced medical sciences or social attitudes in some way.

In other cases, the particular timing of certain plagues – or the quick-thinking of individuals who took advantage of that timing – resulted in major shifts in the tides of wars or in the control of lands and peoples. A particularly famous example is the Spanish conquest of modern-day Mexico. Hernán Cortés, one of the conquistadors who began the Spanish colonization of the Americas, with fewer than six hundred men, managed to conquer the entirety of the Aztec Empire, which comprised millions of citizens. This conquest, along with Francisco Pizarro's conquest of the Inca Empire that soon followed, resulted in the near-complete disappearance of the Mexican and Peruvian native religions and cultures, as millions of native peoples were either killed or converted to Christianity. Though Cortés might tell you that his overwhelming victory had everything to do with his own military might and cunning mind, more likely, it had a great deal to do with an epidemic of smallpox that broke out among the Aztecs only a few months after they successfully drove Cortés from their city. This disease, likely brought to the Americas by the Europeans, struck a population which had no prior exposure to it, and thus lacked the inherited or acquired resistances to combat it. The plague was utterly devastating, killing nearly a third of the Aztec population.

According to Canadian historian William H. McNeill, the psychological implications of this event are just as significant as the massive death toll in the success of Cortés' conquest – the plague killed only Aztecs, leaving the Spanish invaders unharmed. We now understand that the lopsided impact of the disease was a result of the immunity the Europeans had built up through previous exposure to smallpox, but at the time, this evident biological favoritism towards the Spanish could only be interpreted as supernatural; it displayed the overt superiority of the God worshipped by the conquerors over the native gods and religions of the Aztecs. The widespread impact of infectious diseases upon Indigenous American populations offers a key to understanding the ease with which Europe conquered the Americas, both militarily and culturally. When we think about global historical conquests, we often think about military might and strategy – we do not often consider, in the words of McNeill, "the history of humanity's encounters with infectious diseases, and the far-reaching consequences that ensued whenever contacts across disease boundaries allowed a new infection to invade a population that lacked any acquired immunity to its ravages."[6]

Notable Mentions

There are several pandemics we were unable to examine for our book, most notably Tuberculosis, Zika Virus, and AIDS. This omission by no means reflects the relative importance of those pandemics, but is simply a product of our time and size constraints. The following paragraphs will provide a brief overview of those diseases.

Tuberculosis (TB) is a serious and infectious disease caused by the bacterium Mycobacterium tuberculosis, and it is spread between people through airborne droplets released through coughs and sneezes. The disease has likely been in existence for millions of years, but the term 'tuberculosis' was only coined in

---

6   McNeill 1998: 19-21.

1834 by Johann Schoenlein.[7] TB primarily affects the lungs and can cause symptoms such as a prolonged cough, chest pain, weakness and fatigue, fever, or weight loss. Symptoms usually remain mild for several months which can prevent patients from seeking medical care, thus increasing the risk that the infection will spread. Most patients contract TB in its latent form, which causes no symptoms and cannot be passed on to others.[8] Tuberculosis cases began to increase in the 1980s, largely attributed to emerging HIV epidemics. The HIV virus weakens an individual's immune system and makes it very difficult for the body to fight disease, particularly TB. In fact, tuberculosis is the leading cause of death in HIV patients. Although tuberculosis is curable (through a six month course of four antibiotics), the disease causes 1.5 million deaths every year, and over 10 million cases.[9] Approximately half of these cases are found in China, Bangladesh, India, Indonesia, Pakistan, Nigeria, the Philippines, and South Africa, but tuberculosis can appear anywhere across the globe. The disease has been known to mutate into drug resistant strains, and this makes treatment more difficult. Due to its treatable nature, the UN has announced plans to eradicate TB by 2030 through their Sustainable Development Goals, and reported TB cases continue to fall by approximately two percent every year. Promisingly, 58 million lives have been saved between 2000 and 2018 due to accurate tuberculosis diagnosis and treatment.[10]

The Zika virus has appeared around the world throughout different time periods and has caused serious damage to various populations. The first case of the virus was discovered in monkeys in 1947, while the first human case was reported in the African

---

7   Barberis, Bragazzi, Galluzzo, & Martini, 2017.

8   Mayo Clinic, n.d.

9   WHO, 2020.

10 Ibid.

countries of Uganda and Tanzania in 1952. If a person were to contract the virus, they would start exhibiting symptoms as early as three days or as late as fourteen days. Fortunately, the World Health Organization reported that the majority of those who did contract the virus did not exhibit any symptoms, and if they did, these symptoms were mild. Some of the common symptoms, which typically last around a week, are fever, rash, muscle pain, and headache. The virus is transmitted through Aedes mosquitoes which primarily reside in tropical countries, where many of the Zika virus outbreaks have occurred. The first ever reported outbreak occurred in 2007 in Yap island, a part of Micronesia. The most recent outbreak of the virus occurred in 2015, originating in Brazil. The major problem associated with the Zika virus is the potential complications that arise from the disease. Unfortunately, if a pregnant person contracts the disease, the virus can be transmitted to the fetus. This could result in the loss of the fetus or to a stillbirth. Two specific diseases that may occur if a pregnant person contracts the disease are Guillain-Barré syndrome and microcephaly. Guillain-Barré syndrome results in the immune system fighting the body's own nervous system, while microcephaly leads to reduced head size in infants. Both of these diseases result in neurological problems in the infants and could potentially lead to death. There is no official treatment as of yet to counter the Zika virus, but healthcare officials recommend staying hydrated and going on a regular course of antibiotics.[11]

The AIDS (acquired immunodeficiency syndrome) pandemic began in 1981 with an outbreak of infections in homosexual men in New York and California. The key symptom of this disease was a complete deficiency in CD4+ lymphocytes, which would increase a person's susceptibility to other diseases and infections.[12] HIV (human immunodeficiency virus) was later determined to be the

---

11   WHO, 2018.
12   Piot and Quinn, 2013.

cause of AIDS. Within a year, AIDS had also been identified in hemophiliacs, injecting drug users, blood transfusion recipients and infants of affected mothers. AIDS is spread through activities that involve bodily fluid transfer, such as sex and sharing needles. AIDS spread to Africa and Asia during the 1980's. By the mid-1990's, fatalities began decreasing due to the development of antiretroviral drugs.[13] The main prevention methods for AIDS are the use of condoms during sex and the use of sterile equipment for injections and bloodwork. However, it can be hard to promote safe sex and injections due to the private nature of these two activities, especially with the continued prevalence of illicit drugs. The wide spread of AIDS spurred a global response, including a Declaration of Commitment on HIV/AIDS by the WHO that was created in 2001 and renewed in 2011. The AIDS pandemic is similar to our COVID-19 crisis in numerous ways: both diseases are caused by zoonotic viruses, both infections have spread on a global scale, and there are currently no available vaccines for either disease. There are still millions of people living with HIV/AIDS to this day, but improved treatment and prevention options are steadily reducing case numbers.

    This book is arranged chronologically, with the first chapter concerning a plague from the 2nd century AD, and the final chapters detailing what is currently known about the present, on-going pandemic that is COVID-19, followed by a discussion on the global future of pandemics. Each chapter will discuss an individual plague or pandemic and present it in the context of its unique time and place. The significance and scale of each pandemic, as well as how the people of its time understood and dealt with the disease, will ideally, by the end of the book, allow the reader to understand the current effects and impact of COVID-19 within its proper historical context. Learning how our predecessors responded and reacted when confronted with

---

13   Ibid.

similar events in the past helps us both understand and better prepare for present and future challenges.

Chapter 1: Antonine Plague (165-180)

Alex Elvidge

> "This pestilence must have raged with incredible fury; and it carried off innumerable victims. As the reign of M. Aurelius forms a turning point in so many things, and above all in literature and art, I have no doubt that this crisis was brought about by that plague. ...The ancient world never recovered from the blow inflicted upon it by the plague which visited it in the reign of M. Aurelius."
> - Barthold Georg Nieburh (1776-1831)[14]

In the mid-2nd century AD, the Roman army, under the leadership of co-emperor Lucius Verus, conducted a war against the Parthian Empire over the regions of Armenia and Upper Mesopotamia. This five-year long war was coming to its end in the winter of 165/166 when the Roman army successfully sieged the Mesopotamian city of Seleucia, located on the Tigris River near modern Baghdad. With Rome's now-inevitable victory in his sights, Emperor Verus was unaware that his army had just stumbled upon a new, unanticipated enemy – a highly infectious disease that would come to wreak havoc and death over the entirety of the Roman Empire.

The Antonine Plague, named for Verus' co-emperor, Marcus Aurelius Antoninus, ravaged the Roman Empire from 165 to 180 AD. Though there is no way to know for certain where the virus actually began, it is undeniable that the Roman army's siege of Seleucia was the event that ignited the plague's rapid, relentless spread across the empire. Roman historians of the 4th century

---
14 Niebuhr 1849: 251.

evidently believed that the plague was the result of Roman sacrilege and the violation of a divine sanctuary. The biography of Verus from the collection of imperial lives Scriptores Historiae Augustae tells us that the virus arose after a temple of Apollo in Seleucia was plundered and its statue stolen, upon which time a spiritus pestilens (a pestilent or infected spirit) was released.[15] The virus first spread among the Parthians, and then, once it infected the Roman army, followed Verus all the way back to Rome, and then spread north and west, to the Rhine and to Gaul and to the rest of the empire.

In the 2nd century, the Roman Empire had the finest and most efficient military force the world had ever seen. The army maintained such a degree of peace in the empire that the 2nd century historian Tacitus bemoaned the fact that there were no great wars to write about in his time. It is all the more ironic, therefore, that the degree and vastness of devastation wrought by the Antonine Plague was in large part due to the Roman army. As with the 1918 flu pandemic, soldiers returning home from the front were largely responsible for facilitating the spread of the disease. The Roman army – a massive, constantly moving force – carried the disease from place to place, to large cities and small villages that had never before faced such a blight and were unequipped to handle it.

After the siege of Seleucia, large numbers of troops succumbed to the disease as imperial forces continued to move east under the command of Emperor Verus. Many towns and villages in the Italian Peninsula and European provinces were left without a single living inhabitant, as those who were not killed by the plague were forced to flee in order to escape infection. As the disease spread north to the Roman legions stationed along the Rhine, it infected Germanic and Gallic peoples outside the borders of the empire. These northern groups had been slowly

---

15 Scriptores Historiae Augustae, Verus 8.1-2; Rolfe 1940: 363.

moving south over the past several years in search of more lands to sustain their growing populations. With the Roman army considerably thinned by the epidemic, they were now unable to continue to push the northern tribes back. Emperor Marcus Aurelius personally commanded the legions near the Danube to try to control the advance of the Germanic peoples across the river. He was forced to concede to allow the Germanic tribes to settle in the frontier provinces of the empire.

Galen and Smallpox

Many today are familiar with the name Galen, at the time known as Claudius Galenus, a Greek physician from the 2nd century whose impressive volume of writings formed the foundation of medical knowledge and practice in Europe and the Islamic world until the 16th century. Along with Hippocrates (of "Hippocratic Oath" fame), Galen is one of the most well-known medical writers of antiquity. The Antonine Plague holds an important place in the history of medicine because of its association with this particular physician.

Galen was in Rome when the plague reached the city in 166 AD, and was present at an outbreak among the Roman troops stationed at Aquileia in the winter of 168/169. Much of what we know about the symptoms of the Antonine Plague come from Galen's writings on his experience observing and treating these soldiers. Unfortunately, though Galen wrote with great detail on several other diseases and their methods of treatment, his descriptions of the Antonine Plague are brief and incomplete. Unlike Thucydides' account of the Athenian plague over 600 years earlier, Galen had no interest in providing a detailed description of the disease so that it could be recognized by later generations should a future outbreak occur. If he had, perhaps the second outbreak that did occur 24 years later would have been less devastating.

Spread and Symptoms

Galen called the Antonine Plague "a fever plague". Based on his descriptions of the physical effects of the disease, scholars have tentatively diagnosed the plague as either smallpox, exanthematous typhus or bubonic plague, with smallpox being the preferred diagnosis. Smallpox is a respiratory virus, therefore it is spread mostly by breathing and coughing. It is also what is referred to as a "crowd disease" – in order for the virus to successfully establish itself within a population, there has to be enough people in close enough contact with one another for the disease to be transmitted and maintained. If the population is too small, the disease will blow through it and fade away fairly immediately – smallpox kills quickly, and a virus without a host cannot survive. Thus, it is no coincidence that smallpox began spreading globally just as human population size took off with the development of farming and the agricultural revolution.

Smallpox has an incubation period – the amount of time between when you're infected and when you start to show symptoms – of 10 to 12 days. With many viruses, the infected individual can still be contagious during the incubation period, which is typically what leads to such wide spread of the disease, as individuals who show no symptoms and do not know they are infected continue to infect others. However, smallpox is not quite so sneaky – it does not tend to be infectious until the patient starts to show symptoms, with your most infectious period being when you have some of more severe symptoms. However, smallpox can be relentless – once recovered, people develop immunity to the disease for an extended period of time, with the result that each new wave of the highly infectious epidemic sweeps primarily through the children who are born in the interim.

If you were a citizen of the Roman Empire in the mid to late 2nd century AD and you contracted the Antonine Plague, here are some of the symptoms you might have experienced:

First, you would develop a severe fever. You would experience stomach pains, likely vomiting, and foul breath with an insatiable thirst. Next, diarrhea – this would start out auburn colored, then become yellowish-red, and later black. Diarrhea was an inseparable symptom of the disease and suffered by all, whether they ultimately survived the plague or died from it.

Somewhere between the seventh and the eleventh day, you might experience blackish stool. If your stool was very dark black, this would indicate gastrointestinal bleeding, which meant you were very likely going to die. If, however, the stool was not black, and if you lived to the ninth day, your entire body would become covered in skin breakouts, similar to a pimpled rash, which could be either dry or pustular, in raised blisters. If you were lucky, a black rash would appear over your whole body, which in most cases would be ulcerated and dry, with no liquid oozing out. If you reached this point, you would likely live to see the other side of this disease. This blackness would be due to the blood which had putrified in the fever blisters, and was a sign of the illness having mostly passed. These blisters would eventually scab and when the scab would fall away, healthy skin would remain beneath, and after one or two days, this would scar over.

You might perhaps develop a cough around day nine. By the tenth day, the cough would become stronger, and would be accompanied by a back-up of mucus in the nose and throat. After suffering this cough for several days, you would begin to cough up blood. If you coughed up scabs (as opposed to fresh blood), this might be an indication of an ulcerated area in the windpipe and an infected larynx, from which you might suffer permanent vocal damage.

If you survived to the twelfth day, you would likely be able to get out of bed.

Impact

Emperor Marcus Aurelius was the last of five great emperors whose combined efforts raised the Roman Empire to an unprecedented pinnacle of power and prosperity in the 2nd century. Historian Edward Gibbon describes this period as "the happiest and most prosperous period" in the history of the human race.3[16] In 165 AD, the Roman Empire was at its height – some would say the plague marked the onset of a century of decline. It occurred in the midst of a series of important wars that challenged Roman supremacy, and the combination of war and disease likely had a significant impact on the weakening of the Roman state. Historian Arthur E. R. Boak argues that the Antonine Plague ignited a period of declining population in the empire, which made maintaining numbers in the Roman army difficult, requiring the increased dependency on non-Roman citizens in the military.[17] Thus, the plague severely impacted Roman military might, as well as Roman culture, literature, and maritime trade relations in the Indian Ocean, severely decreasing Roman commercial activity in Southeast Asia. Barbarian invasions and warfare, economic distress, political instability, famine, and recurrent outbreaks of disease reduced the might of the empire

---

16 Gibbon 1909: 85-6.

17 Boak 1955.

severely by the mid-200s, by which time large portions of the empire in the east and west had broken away. Some historians suggest that the combined effect of the smallpox and malaria viruses – of which there were seasonal outbreaks for hundreds of years – largely contributed to the eventual fall of the Roman Empire.

The Antonine Plague devastated the European population on a scale that had never before been experienced. The first leg of this prolonged and destructive disease lasted until the death of Marcus Aurelius in 180 AD. In these 15 years, the plague racked up a death count in the millions. While earlier scholars, based on the vague and likely exaggerated accounts of ancient sources, estimated that over half the population of the Roman Empire succumbed to the disease,[18] a more conservative picture of the effects of the plague suggests a much smaller, yet still devastating, 2 percent of the population of the empire – 1 million deaths.[19] Most scholars now agree on a reasonable mortality rate of 7 to 10 percent – approximately 3.5 to 5 million deaths.

In any highly contagious pandemic, denser population areas where many people are crowded together, such as cities and army encampments, are usually hardest hit. The entire Roman world was not yet highly urbanized, but still much of the population was clustered in large, congested cities. The mortality rates in such areas and in the Roman army during the Antonine Plague would have been considerably higher than average, perhaps 13 to 15 percent. In some areas, the disease killed roughly one quarter of those who were infected, and in others, as much as one third of the population. Rome was hit particularly hard – the effects of the plague here were devastating, mostly due to crowding and poor sanitary conditions.

Nine years after the death of Marcus Aurelius, in 189 AD during

---

18 Seeck 1910: 398-405.
19 Gilliam 1961: 225-51.

Emperor Commodus' reign, another plague occurred. Dio Cassius, a Roman statesman and historian living at the time, wrote that this plague was the greatest of any of which he had knowledge. It was commonplace for 2,000 deaths to occur per day in Rome alone, as the plague killed humans and livestock alike, and thus was accompanied by a great famine.[20] This is widely assumed to be another outbreak of the Antonine Plague. The entire pandemic therefore lasted for a total of 24 years, with sporadic flare-ups, and the total number of deaths falling somewhere between 7 and 10 million.

No account of the plague currently exists which is comprehensive, precise, and reliable. This lack of accurate or extensive statistical data is to be expected in any study of events from antiquity. Even if we did happen to have reliable statistics for the deaths that occurred in just one city during the Antonine Plague, we would be unable to generalize about the whole empire due to the lack of consistent extant records of the time. However, even if we were to rely on the most conservative estimated mortality count, the Antonine Plague would still be the cause of more deaths than any other epidemic or pandemic to date. A virus to this effect would not be felt again in the Roman Empire until the mid-3rd century.

---

20 Dio Cassius 72.14.3-4.

Chapter 2: The Plague of Justinian (541-549)

Alex Elvidge

"During these times there was a pestilence, by which the whole human race came near to being annihilated...For it did not come in a part of the world nor upon certain men, nor did it confine itself to any season of the year, so that from such circumstances it might be possible to find subtle explanations for a cause, but it embraced the entire world, and blighted the lives of all men..."
- Procopius (mid-6th century AD)[21]

When you think of plague, usually Black Death is one of the first thoughts that come to mind. That 14th century strain of bubonic plague was so devastating and widespread in its destruction that the event came to define our perception of pandemics and infectious diseases, to the point where the words "Black Death" have become, in essence, synonymous with plague itself. But the 14th century was not the first time that Yersinia pestis, the infectious bacterium responsible for the bubonic plague, made its way into Europe. In fact, you would have to travel back eight centuries before the events of the Black Death, to 541 AD, in order to experience the first global calamity caused by the deadly bacterium known as Yersinia pestis.

Let's take a step back to define our terms. As you may have noticed, plague has two separate but closely related meanings in the context of virulent disease – there's plague, and there's plague. When we say "the plague", typically we are referring to the particular infectious disease caused by the bacterium Yersinia

---
21   Procopius, History of the Wars, Book II, 22.1-7.

pestis, which is spread from rats to humans by means of flea bites. The Black Death was this type of plague, and it was such an infamous event in our history that it has come to define our idea of what a plague can actually be. However, we don't use plague just to refer to the disease caused by Yersinia pestis. More broadly, plague can simply refer to any epidemic or pandemic disease that causes high mortality - think pestilence.[22] Used figuratively, plague can also refer to any widespread calamity or evil - think biblical plagues. You may have asked yourself – is the coronavirus a plague? Yes and no. It is not the plague, since COVID-19 is caused by a virus, whereas the plague is caused by bacteria. However, the coronavirus is a plague, in the sense that it is a highly infectious disease that is causing widespread affliction. For the sake of clarity, when this book discusses the three historical outbreaks of the plague caused by the bacterium Yersinia pestis, it will delineate them as such. Otherwise, when plague is used, it will refer to the broader definition of the word, meaning pestilence.

The Journey of Yersinia pestis

Yersinia pestis is a bacterium endemic to many countries around the world. Three of the most devastating pandemics in human history have been associated with the plague caused by Yersinia pestis. The Plague of Justinian, often referred to as the "first plague pandemic", which began in 541 and persisted in some capacity all the way until 750 AD, was the first recorded outbreak of this particular plague. Named for Justinian, the Eastern Roman Emperor who ruled from 527 to 565 AD, the disease afflicted the

---

[22] Pestilence comes from the Latin pestis, a noun meaning "destruction, disease, plague, ruin". Plague is from the Latin plaga, meaning "wound, affliction, injury, misfortune".

entirety of the Mediterranean Basin, Europe, and the Near East. The plague severely affected not just one dominant world power, but two – the Sasanian Empire, the last pre-Islamic Persian Empire, and the Eastern Roman Empire, which by then was called Byzantium. By this time, the Roman empire had been split up into two separate factions, East and West, and the Western Roman Empire had fallen in the previous century. Emperor Justinian was ruling from the capital of the Eastern Roman Empire, Constantinople, which was particularly devastated by the plague.

The plague purportedly first appeared at Pelusium in Egypt, at the eastern edge of the Nile delta, in 541. It moved west to Alexandria and east to Palestine, and reached Constantinople within just a year. From there, it made its way into North Africa, Italy, Spain, and into the French-German border by the winter of 543. It continued to spread around the Mediterranean Sea until 544, and persisted in Northern Europe and the Arabian Peninsula until 549. Though that year marked the end of the first major wave of the disease, the Plague of Justinian was actually just the start of a 200-year period of recurring epidemics. Scholars have identified between fifteen and seventeen waves of plague between 541 and 767 AD.[23] It is contentious to refer to the Antonine Plagues from several centuries previous as a pandemic – though it did decimate the Roman Empire and what was at the time considered "the known world", it did not reach all major areas of the globe, and for this reason many still refer to it as a large epidemic. The Justinian Plague, meanwhile, can be properly referred to as a pandemic, as it affected vast and numerous global regions in a repeated, lengthy series of outbreaks.

---

23 Stathakopoulos 2000: 256-276; Biraben and LeGoff 1975: 44-80.

The Humble Flea and the Well-Travelled Rat

When it reached the empire's capital in 542, the plague was already headed down an inevitable path of destruction that, by then, was impossible to stop. But how did this disease come to be? Yersinia pestis actually took a rather lengthy and convoluted journey in order to burrow itself into the heart of one of the most powerful empires in history. This plague is a zoonotic disease, meaning it generally circulates in animal populations and occasionally spills over into human populations. Frighteningly, over 200 mammalian species are known to be naturally infected with the bacterium that causes plague, but it is largely endemic in communities of wild rodents, and most commonly reaches humans when it is carried from a rodent by a flea. In order for this disease to take hold, humans must unwittingly do two things: (1) be in close contact with an infected population of rodents and (2) live in places where fleas can flourish as well.

Climate change may have played a significant role in bringing these harbingers of bacteria closer to human populations. Like disease, climate change has been a permanent feature of human existent, far before the age of industrialization. Global temperatures change with variations in the Earth's orbit and solar cycles, and volcanic eruptions spew reflective sulphates into the atmosphere, contributing to global heating. Hotter climates often result in disease-carrying creatures – like rodents and fleas, which thrive in warm, moist environments – spreading to new regions. Due to a number of circumstances during the reign of Justinian, including a series of large volcanic eruptions in the 530s and 540s AD, climate instability seems to have peaked. The onset of the Justinian Plague likely coincided with a very large switch from a drier to a wetter, warmer climate. This change would have led to an unwelcome explosion of rodent and flea populations in urban and rural areas alike.[24]

Before the plague can bring humanity to its knees, the true victim of the disease is actually the humble flea. When a flea bites an infected rat, the bacterium travels to the flea's stomach, where it begins to multiply. Within 3-9 days after taking that infected bite, the flea's bacteria have multiplied so much that they entirely block the esophagus of the flea. The flea becomes so hungry that it tries to bite another rat, but it is unsuccessful because access to its stomach is completely blocked off by the accumulation of bacteria in its esophagus. In order to relieve itself of this blockage, the flea regurgitates a mixture of blood and bacteria into its new rat host. Sadly, the flea will end up dying of starvation and dehydration anyway. But in the new rat, Yersinia pestis will spread from the bite wound into the lymphatic system, where it will replicate and eventually spread to the bloodstream and major organs. This is the general life cycle of the disease, continuing indefinitely when another flea bites this newly infected rat and the process begins again. This process can be contained to rodents and fleas, never infecting humans, at least until a particularly ambitious infected flea decides to bite a human, from which point the bacterium enters the human lymphatic system and often the bloodstream, causing rapid infection.

Since most rodents choose to live their lives in a rather slow, rather sedentary sort of way, the spread of this disease from one place to another depends on humans taking it upon themselves to move these rodents over large distances. Luckily, the rat is a skilled climber, and finds it easy enough to board our ships and laze its way across the ocean, trotting ashore and depositing its bacteria at each new port while we happily ferry it from place to place. Rats originated in the east, so the arrival of these rodents

---

24   Harper 2017.

in the western world was likely the result of the opening of early sea communications between Egypt and India, and in subsequent centuries the rodent-traveller presumably extended its range inland from the ports.

Recent genetic studies of Yersinia pestis DNA suggest that the Justinian Plague originated in Central Asia.[25] However, the geographic origins of the plague are still in dispute, as the historians who lived through the plague believed that it first appeared in Egypt. The intricate trade routes make either origin a possibility, and travel networks were so well established by this point in the empire that regardless of where the disease began, its rapid, destructive spread was inevitable. The period of Justinian was one of very active and extensive commerce, especially by sea. Constantinople, being the capital, had a great demand for foreign goods brought in from all over the known world and would import large amounts of resources from other regions – this, unfortunately, made the city a major point of diffusion for disease. If we are to trust our ancient sources' belief that the plague began in Egypt, it does not take a strong imagination to conceptualize how it might have reached the capital. Egypt was a major source of grain at this time, often sending large ships of their export throughout the empire. The rat and flea population in Egypt was particularly rampant at this time as well (because rodents fed from the large granaries that held the country's primary export), and where there are rodents, there are fleas. When Egypt would send ships of grain across the sea, unwilling to let their food go on without them, the rats would tag along, and it would have only taken one infected rat to carry the plague from Egypt to Constantinople, from which point the disease would have travelled along the trade routes to every major city in the empire.

---

25   Harbeck, M., et al. 2013.

Symptoms

If you were to encounter the bubonic plague today, you would likely be just fine. Unlike with a virus, bacterial infections are easily cured with the help of modern antibiotics, as long as you catch it early enough. However, if you became infected with the plague in the 6th century, you would not have been so lucky – if untreated with antibiotics, the bubonic form of the plague can be fatal in 30-60% of cases. The incubation period for the bubonic plague – the time from when you get infected to when you start showing symptoms – is 1-7 days. Symptoms would strike suddenly with a high fever, chills, head and body aches, vomiting and nausea – fairly standard fare, apart from the characteristic buboes, the bacteria-filled lumps that give the bubonic plague its name. These would appear all over your body – on your groin, armpits, neck, thighs, and behind your ears, and some buboes could grow as large as an apple. Luckily, it is difficult for humans to infect one another with bubonic plague – you would have to have a lot of contact with someone else's bubo in order to get sick yourself. After a few days of being infected with bubonic plague, your buboes would be replaced by black spots, which would spread all over your skin, first few and large, then small and numerous. The advanced stages of bubonic plague could also result in open sores. Within a few days, you might become delirious or slip into a coma, after which time, if you were lucky, you would recover, and if you were unlucky, you wouldn't wake up again.

Not everyone who is infected with the plague has buboes, however – there are two other kinds of plague caused by Yersinia pestis: septicemic, which happens when an overload of bacteria travels from your lymph nodes into your bloodstream, and pneumonic, which occurs in the unlucky few whose bubonic plague has spread to their lungs. The pneumonic form of plague is incredibly contagious and by far the most deadly. It is the most virulent form of the disease as it is transmitted human to human via respiratory droplets, like the flu, like smallpox, and like the coronavirus. It takes over your body very rapidly, in some cases within 24 hours, and if untreated with antibiotics, pneumonic plague is almost 100% fatal.

Impact

The actual number of deaths that resulted from the Justinian Plague is uncertain. Some modern scholars believe the plague killed up to 5,000 people per day in Constantinople at the peak of the pandemic. Though there were frequent subsequent waves of the plague that continued to strike throughout the 6th, 7th, and 8th centuries, with time the disease became less virulent and more localized. Though some evidence exists for the serious impact of the pandemic on the size of the global population, no certain figure exists. Some ancient writers documented outlandish figures – Procopius, Justinian's court historian, suggests that the European population dropped by half due to the pandemic, recording that the plague killed 10,000 people in Constantinople a day.[26] Emperor Justinian was said to have contracted the disease himself at the height of the pandemic, though he eventually recovered.[27] John of Ephesus, another contemporary witness of the pandemic, claims that the total death toll in Constantinople

---

26 Procopius, History of the Wars, Book II, 22.6-39.
27 Procopius, History of the Wars, Book II, 23.19-24.4.

may have been 300,000.[28] Of course, many question the accuracy of such numbers – remember, ancient historians have an interest in a good story, often at the expense of truth and transparency. However, contemporaries did write of villages that were entirely deserted, and recent archaeology has discovered mass burial sites from the period. There was a relative absence of new public buildings constructed in the years after 540 AD, and the creation of new rural settlements also slowed somewhat after that date, indicating an overall diminution of population.

The plague had several immediate as well as long-term effects on the populations and cultures of the European world. Short-term, the economy was a wreck – all work ceased, shops closed for lack of workers and customers, fields were abandoned, and crops went unharvested. The psychological effects on the people of the empire must have been staggering. Procopius notes that because there was not enough room to bury the massive amounts of the dead, bodies were left stacked in the open, and the entire capital smelled like death. The empire allotted public money for digging mass graves – when those were filled, boats were loaded with the dead, whose remains were dumped overboard at sea. People took to wearing name tags on their arms when they left their homes so that they might be identified if they should die suddenly while they were out.[29]

The wide-reaching impact of the plague on the progression of European and Christian history was great as well. Some scholars believe that the social, economic, cultural, and political effects of this plague's disruption may have contributed to the transition between the ancient and medieval periods of Western

---

28 Unfortunately, John of Ephesus' original writings survive only in fragments. He wrote the longest known account of the Justinian Plague in part 2 of his Chronicle, which is now lost, but was quoted extensively in the writings of Pseudo-Dionysius of Tel-Mahre at the end of the 8th century.

29 Procopius, History of the Wars, Book II, 23.4-19.

history.[30] Before the plague hit, Justinian had been in the middle of a massive multi-front conquest in the name of re-uniting the empire, and he was winning. Justinian's armies were just about to retake all of Italy and the western Mediterranean coast, and the conquest would likely have successfully restored the unity of Roman Empire. However, the plague struck at a critical point – the conflict with the Goths was waning, but as the disease spread to port cities around the Mediterranean, the struggling Goths were reinvigorated and their conflict with Constantinople entered a new phase. In 568, the Lombards invaded Northern Italy and defeated the small Byzantine army that had been left behind and established the Kingdom of the Lombards. Indeed, Justinian's failure to restore unity to the Mediterranean under the empire can be attributed in large part to the diminution of imperial resources stemming from the plague. Some scholars go so far as to say that the major cultural changes that occurred in the following centuries, such as the rise of Islam, the growing divergence between eastern and western Christianity, and the progressive localization of the economies, political systems, and societies of western Europe, were all aided or accelerated by the persistent epidemic disasters that occurred between the 6th and 8th centuries.

---

30   Russell 1968: 174-184.

Chapter 3: The Black Death (1346-1353)

Alex Elvidge

"The 'burn blisters' appeared, and boils developed in different parts of the body: on the sexual organs, in others on the thighs, or on the arms, and in others on the neck. At first these were the size of a hazelnut and the patient was seized by violent shivering fits, which soon rendered him so weak that he could no longer stand upright [...] Soon the boils grew to the size of a walnut, then to that of a hen's egg or a goose's egg, and they were exceedingly painful [...] The blood rose from the affected lungs to the throat, producing a putrefying and ultimately decomposing effect on the whole body. The sickness lasted three days, and on the fourth, at the latest, the patient succumbed."
- Michael of Piazza, Franciscan chronicler of the Black Death at Messina in 1347[31]

The Crisis of the Late Middle Ages

The late Middle Ages were far from a peaceful and prosperous time in human history. Death was a common occurrence, with frequent wars, natural disasters, diseases, and poor living conditions being constant companions. The early 14th-century was a particularly bad time in Europe, with a series of large-scale crises striking the continent in quick succession. Prior to this point, Europe had experienced several centuries of relative stability – the 13th century had been a period of economic

---

31   Scott and Duncan 2004: 14-15.

expansion and urbanization, and demographic growth had doubled the European population between 1100 and 1300 AD. However, this positive growth and development did not remain so; as substantial towns with populations upwards of fifteen thousand and growing began to pop up around Europe, crowding and unsanity housing became more significant issues. This massive population growth coincided with several successive years of bad weather: torrential rain, widespread flooding, windstorms, and brutal winters followed by summers with unseasonably cool temperatures that shortened the growing season. What resulted was a series of catastrophic crop failures, leading to a period of social and economic hardship. The economic recession produced lower wages and contributed to growing poverty, which in turn caused agricultural production to fall even further. In short, population growth was exceeding output – Europe was gearing up for a famine.

The late medieval "Great Famine" lasted from 1315 to 1322 and caused the death of millions across the entire European continent. Children suffered severe malnourishment which led to their becoming immunocompromised in their adulthood.[32] This crisis, devastating in its own right, set the stage for an unfortunate equation when once again, the deadly bacterium Yersinia pestis would decide to make an appearance on Europe's shores. The result of the famine, unsurprisingly, was that resistance to disease was severely compromised among the general populace. When the plague would once again strike the European world less than a quarter-century later, it would be nothing less than the deadliest pandemic ever recorded in human history.

The Black Death, as the second plague pandemic would come to be known, was once of the worst humanitarian disasters the world had ever seen. Though much of the global population had

---

32   Snowden 2019: 37.

already been exposed to the bacterium Yersinia pestis, this time, it would kill twice as many people, and would irrevocably alter nations and cultures and the way we respond to outbreaks of disease. But why was Yersinia pestis so much more devastating the second time around? One would think that those populations that had endured previous exposure to the disease during the Plague of Justinian would have developed a degree of immunity, as with the Europeans who were resistant to the Smallpox that decimated the Aztec Empire during the Spanish colonization of the Americas. However, genetic findings have demonstrated that the strain of Yersinia pestis that caused the Plague of Justinian was genetically distant from the strains responsible for the second and third plague pandemics – it mutated. Therefore, the population was unable to develop to develop any resistance to the plague – it was as if they were fighting a completely new disease. This factor, along with the aforementioned surrounding crises in the late Middle Ages that combined to generally weaken the immune systems of the European populace, helps explain the extraordinary virulence and rapid spread of the Black Death.

The Second Journey of Yersinia pestis

The Plague of Justinian, discussed in the previous chapter, is considered the first plague pandemic. The second plague pandemic began sometime in the 1330s, reached the Western World in 1347, and persisted with varying severity for centuries, until the plague finally disappeared in the 1830s. Though we tend to think of the Black Death as synonymous with "the plague", when we say "Black Death" we actually are referring only to the first European wave of the second plague pandemic, which occurred from 1347 until 1353.

The Black Death likely originated in Central or East Asia and travelled along the Silk Road, a network of trade routes which connected the Eastern and Western worlds. The road derives its name from the lucrative silk trade that it facilitated, and was a pathway at the center of most economic, cultural, political, and religious interactions for nearly 2000 years. The Silk Road was largely responsible for the disease spreading so quickly and over such a vast area of the world. Also to blame was sea trade – as with the Plague of Justinian, the bacterium was carried over large distances by fleas living on the infected rats that travelled on ships. Once it reached the shore, the disease was spread to humans by those fleas. Some scholars attribute the incredibly rapid spread of the Black Death to human to human transmission. If the bacterium infects the lungs, the plague becomes pneumonic, and thus can be spread through respiratory droplets or aerosols when we talk, breath, or cough too close to someone else. The pneumonic form of the plague is the most virulent form of the disease and would explain how the Black Death spread so rapidly, and how it killed so quickly.

The pandemic is conventionally thought to have arrived in Europe aboard Genoese merchant ships sailing from the Black Sea in the summer of 1347. These merchant vessels crossed into the Mediterranean Basin, Africa, Western Asia, and the rest of Europe via Constantinople, Sicily, and the Italian Peninsula, depositing the bacterium at each location. When the Genoese ships docked at Messina in Sicily, the disease is thought to have spread rapidly to Sardinia and Corsica, and then somewhat more slowly to mainland Italy, and onwards from there to the whole of Europe. In individual places the outbreak usually lasted about three or four months, and much of the death toll occurred in that brief span. At this time, Italy was very active at the center of Mediterranean trade. It is therefore no coincidence that the Italian cities were the first in Europe to be hit hard by the plague as they facilitated the import and export of resources from all over the world.

Symptoms

The symptoms of the 14th century plague were much the same as the symptoms of the 6th century plague. Both were characterized by dark buboes covering the whole body and gangrene of the extremities. This necrosis of the nose, fingers, and toes is supposedly what gave the Black Death its name. High fever, shivering, violent headaches, nausea, vomiting, and terrible thirst are all symptoms of the first phase of the disease. The second phase is primarily about the buboes – according to 16th-century French surgeon Ambroise Paré, the bubo generated great heat and caused a burning and prickling, needle-like pain.[33] What's more, all of the regular bodily excretions – urine, sweat, breath, pus – developed an overpowering and intolerable stench.

If you were sick with the bubonic plague and the multiplying Yersinia pestis bacteria in your system were to gain access to your bloodstream, they would release a powerful toxin that would likely be fatal. The toxin causes the degeneration of the tissues of the heart, liver, spleen, kidneys, lungs, and central nervous system – what is known as multiple organ failure. At this point in the disease, you might have bloodshot eyes, a black tongue, and a pale face, and you would not have much control of your facial muscles. You would also have progressive neurological damage, which would manifest itself in slurred speech, leg and arm tremors, a staggering gait, seizures, and delirium resulting in either coma or death. If you were fortunate enough to recover from your ordeal, you would likely face some permanent

---
33 Cunningham and Grell 2000: 283.

physiological damage: deafness, impaired vision, paralysis of one or more limbs, inability to speak as a result of laryngeal paralysis, and loss of memory – not to mention the psychological trauma.

Impact

What you'll often hear when you learn about the Black Death is that it "reduced the population of Europe by half". As we've learned in each chapter thus far, these larger numbers are often exaggerated. Especially with the series of crises that was already ravaging Europe at the time the plague struck, it is difficult to separate the mortality rate of the Black Death from the deaths caused by the Great Famine and by every other major and minor disaster that was wreaking havoc on the continent during the late Middle Ages. It is true that it took until around 1500 AD for the European population to regain the demographic levels it reached in 1300. Many historians will say that during its seemingly relentless progress across Europe, the Black Death outstripped even the Great Famine in its impact. However, the famine essentially primed the European population to be annihilated by the plague by decreasing overall immunity to disease. Therefore, any number attributed to the Black Death has to give at least some credit to the famine. It is thus difficult to isolate the death toll of the pandemic alone.

Today's historians have widely come to accept a total mortality between 30 and 40 percent of the European population between 1346 and 1353 – still an unthinkable amount. However, a 2004 review of the Black Death argues that those numbers may be too low. This research indicates that the death toll may be closer to 60% across Europe, with some variation between different economic groups and regions.[34] This number is not completely out of the realm of possibility – plague sufferers often received little to no medical attention. In the early waves of the Black Death, societies were utterly unprepared for what they would face. There were no administrative, medical, or religious facilities in place to cope with the amount of disease and death. Physicians themselves were virtually powerless to treat this supposedly new, fast-acting affliction, and to make matters worse, their profession exposed them disproportionately to risk of infection – doctors were dying in great numbers. If this larger estimate of mortality is correct, it would mean 50 million Europeans died in the 6 or 7 years of the Black Death, out of a population of 80 million. However, outbreaks of the plague continued to occur around the world until the early 19th century. The total number of deaths caused by Yersinia pestis in our history is likely incalculable, and near unimaginable.

What Caused It?

There were many different theories put forward at the time of the Black Death to try to make sense of the degree of destruction caused by the disease. The dominant belief at the time was the miasma theory,[35] which held that diseases such as cholera, chlamydia, and the Black Death were caused by a noxious form of bad air. More often however, the way people of the Middle Ages were able to rationalize such a formidable enemy wreaking such purposeless havoc upon the world was through religion. Muslim religious scholars understood the pandemic as a "martyrdom and

---

34   Benedictow 2004.

35   From μίασμα, the ancient Greek world for "pollution" or, more figuratively, "defilement". Dols 1977: 23.

mercy" from God – if you were a believer, and you survived the disease, it was because God had saved you. If a believer perished from the disease, it was because they had become a martyr and were being gifted with a place in paradise. If you were a non-believer, perishing from the disease was clearly a punishment for your sin. Some Muslim doctors even cautioned against trying to prevent or treat the plague, as it was so clearly sent by God.[36]

The predominant modern theory for the cause of the Black Death, unsurprisingly, has a more scientific foundation. Due to climate change occurring in Asia at the time, rodents began to flee the dry grasslands to more highly populated areas where they would have more reliable sources of food, thus spreading the disease to cities.[37] From there, poor hygiene took over as an incredibly effective transmitter of bacteria. Streets in the medieval period were commonly filthy, humans lived in close contact with live animals and, by extension, various parasites, easily facilitating the spread of transmissible disease. The spread of the plague was even more rampant in poorer areas, where decent sanitation was even more inaccessible and crowding was heightened. Once again, the agricultural revolution and the thousands-year-old human decision to survive together in groups became our downfall.

In many respects, the plague and the Black Death in particular represented the worst imaginable catastrophe. It is no coincidence that we still use the word "plague" to mean any kind of calamity or trouble, whether medical or metaphorical. The plague set the standard by which all past and future epidemics would be judged. In later centuries, when societies would experience outbreaks of new, unfamiliar diseases, they would wait anxiously to see whether these diseases would equal the

---

36 Dols 1977: 23.
37 Tignor et al. 2014: 407.

Black Death in their devastation. Because of its recurring cycles, with a new outbreak every generation, the plague transformed the demographics of early modern Europe. Because of how the Black Death coincided with the after-effects of the Great Famine, the disease afflicted not just the young and the old and the infirm, but people in the prime of their health. It therefore caused a major halt in population growth between the 14th and 18th centuries and had devastating effects on the economy and societal development. But the plague did not only have a negative impact. One early medical advancement that came about as a result of the Black Death was the establishment of the idea of quarantine in 1377, which was employed for the first time after continuing outbreaks in Ragusa (modern Dubrovnik) in Croatia.[38] What's more, the plague substantially influenced religion and popular culture, giving rise to a new genre of art and literature centered around the disease and its psychological impact. Indeed, the Black Death is one of the best examples of an event that affects every aspect of society, in unforeseeable ways both negative and positive.

---

38   Sehdev 2002: 1071-2.

Chapter 4: Smallpox

Mya Colwell

Introduction

Today the word 'smallpox' does not inspire the same fear that it did for thousands of years, and has been reduced to a chapter, albeit a rather long chapter, in history. This deadly disease plagued communities for nearly 3000 years before its eradication in 1979, and terrified people all over the globe due to its grisly symptoms and relentless progression.[39] It wasn't only the young and the old susceptible to smallpox, but anyone who had not been previously exposed to the disease. Peasants, merchants and monarchs succumbed to its pustule encrusted clutches, and children were not officially considered part of the family (for inheritance reasons) until they had survived the disease. Entire populations were decimated, and disease could kill as many as one third of its victims.

Symptoms

Smallpox is an illness caused by either of the two Variola Virus strains: Variola Major and Variola Minor. In unvaccinated patients Variola Major could have a 40-50% mortality rate, although it tended to hover around 20%. Variola Minor on the other hand, had a mortality rate less than 1%.[40] One positive aspect of the virus is that patients were immune to smallpox

---

[39] Kotar, 2013.
[40] Dumbel, Rossier, & Rossier, 1961.

once they had survived it. They could not contract it a second time. COVID-19 has an estimated case-fatality rate of 1.6% in Canada and 1.78% in the United States (as of April 22, 2020).[41] Smallpox was spread similarly to COVID-19: through face-to-face contact between individuals, and droplets transmitted through coughing and sneezing.[42] This occurred in smallpox because the virus was present in scabs and pustules which first appeared on the mouth and throat before progressing to the rest of the body. The disease could also have been transmitted by handling contaminated clothing and bedding. Smallpox symptoms were very similar to those of the Antonine plague discussed in chapter two, and there were several symptoms that preceded the onset of the disease including red eyes; sore throat; pain in the head, loins, and back; weariness and faintness; hot and cold flashes; thirst; nausea; and a quick pulse. Three or four days after these symptoms occurred, small red spots would appear on the face, neck, and breast, usually accompanied by a fever. The spots increased in size for three to four more days to become pustules, and eventually covered the whole body. At this point the face would swell until the eyes shut. On the eleventh day, the swelling in the face, hands and feet would go down and the pustules broke, eventually drying out and falling off in crusts. Smallpox was usually fatal between the eighth and eleventh day, but in some cases, victims perished between the fourteenth and sixteenth day.[43] Those who survived these painful two weeks were left with potential internal organ damage, scars from the large pits left by pustules, and even blindness.

---

41   Abdollahi, Champredon, Langley, Galvani, & Moghadas, 2020.
42   Centers for Disease Control and Prevention.
43   Kotar, 2013.

The Spread of Smallpox

Smallpox has likely been in existence for over 3000 years. The World Health Organization (WHO) offers several theories as to how it came into existence: early humans contracted the virus from rodents after which it mutated into a variola only transmittable to humans, or early humans contracted a "proto-variola" that evolved into smallpox.[44] Although the disease was initially well contained, exploration, religious missions, as well as global population growth soon ensured that the disease was carted across the globe. Heavily populated cities were at a greater risk for smallpox epidemics due to the high turnover of people, and the presence of traders, merchants, soldiers, and slaves. There were more people who were potential carriers of the disease, and the tight quarters increased the likelihood that infected individuals would come into contact with those who had no immunity to the disease.

Smallpox slowly made its way around the globe. After claiming Europe, one of the first places the disease infiltrated was North America. It likely gained entry through the Spanish explorers who landed on the island of Hispaniola in 1507. Hernan Cortez invaded Mexico in 1519, and conquered the Aztec empire in 1521, largely aided by the smallpox he unwittingly brought with him. The disease decimated the Aztec civilization, killing, by some accounts, as many as one third of the Aztec people.[45] The disease progressed through the Valley of Mexico and into Tenochtitlan, then into Guatemala and the Yucatan Peninsula. Smallpox reached the Incan Empire between 1524 and 1527, killing 200,000 of six million Incans and leaving them vulnerable to Spanish conquistador Francisco Pizarro's attacks. Smallpox was introduced

---

44   Ibid
45   Brooks, 1993.

to South America in 1555, and by 1588 the entire continent was inundated with smallpox. Indigenous populations in Canada and the United States were introduced to smallpox in a similar manner to the Aztecs and they had no previous immunity to the disease. Many communities were subsequently decimated after smallpox was introduced by pioneers and settlers, and these pioneers would bring the disease further inland. Major smallpox outbreaks began in 1617 in the United States, while the disease was first introduced to Canada by French settlers in 1635. The disease quickly spread to the Algonquins, Hurons, and other tribes inhabiting New France.

In a twist of fate, subsequent generations of settlers carrying smallpox to the Americas were left unprotected from the disease – a fact that wasn't completely realized until the sons of wealthy landowners traveled to Europe. Cold was no barrier to smallpox, and the disease became fully established in Russia in 1623. Five years later, England would have its first major smallpox outbreak. The slave trade was a driving force behind the transmission of smallpox to Africa, and the first major outbreaks occurred in 1713 in Cape Town. Smallpox was subsequently transmitted into Cuba, Puerto Rico, the Caribbean Islands and Mexico, where slaves were sold. Smallpox was introduced to Greenland in 1734, claiming approximately two thirds of the population, and Iceland suffered from smallpox epidemics in 1797, which killed 18,000 of 50,000 inhabitants. By the 18th century, smallpox was considered to be a major epidemic, especially after its introduction to the previously unaffected Australia in 1789. Ethiopia and Sudan were hit hard with six epidemics of smallpox throughout the 19th century, and the disease continued to be endemic in many countries through to the beginning of the 20th century.[46]

---

46   Theves, Crubezy & Biagini, 2016.

From Magic Lozenges to Vaccination

Smallpox was initially treated with a healthy dose of superstition and a fair amount of pseudoscience. The disease was thought to be caused by miasmas (terrible odours or 'bad air'), and experts recommended purifying the house of noxious smells and preventing the spread of the miasma to other households.[47] In Japan, those ill with smallpox hung red portraits of Tametomo, a 12th century hero rumored to have defeated the smallpox demon, in their bedrooms. The colour red soon became associated with preventing scarring from smallpox, and warding off the worst of the symptoms. Even Queen Elizabeth I spent her smallpox illness (1562) wrapped in a red blanket. This superstition persisted into the late 1930s. Countless tonics and 'miracle cures' set out to proclaim their extraordinary qualities, including Mr. Theophilus Buckworth's "Pectorall Lozenges" which claimed to cure anything from a common cough to smallpox.[48]

Focus turned to discovering a reliable cure, and inoculation (also known as variolation) was introduced to England in the early 1700's by a woman named Lady Mary Wortley Montagu.[49] She had observed inoculation in Constantinople, and enlisted the help of Dr. Maitland to introduce the practice to the British public. Thanks to her considerable patronage, he opened a practice and offered inoculation to the British. She also gained the support of Robert Mead, a prominent physician who wrote several treatises on the subject.

Inoculation was surprisingly effective, and involved inserting a needle into an eruption of smallpox, and injecting that material under the skin of a healthy person. The patient would develop

---

47 Halliday, 2001
48 Kotar, 2013.
49 Ibid.

a mild case of smallpox, and emerge immune to the disease. However, this method was not without its risks. The mild case of smallpox could occasionally develop into a full blown case, and kill the patient. As well, inoculation made patients who survived the procedure carriers of the disease, and capable of infecting healthy people. Therefore, inoculation only worked seamlessly if entire towns and cities underwent the procedure. When done correctly, inoculation did considerably lessen the number of smallpox cases in Europe. The Dublin Journal printed in 1769 that 40,000 people had been inoculated with no more than one hundred perishing from the procedure, and documentation from a charitable hospital at Pancras (outskirts of London) inoculated 1,800 people over several years and only lost eight patients.[50]

Despite Lady Montagu's best efforts, inoculation was met with stringent opposition: religious leaders were against the procedure, claiming that it was a blasphemous attempt to "interrupt the eternal decrees of Providence" and that "all who infused with the variolous ferment were sorcerers, and that inoculation was the diabolical intervention of Satan".[51]

People may also have been concerned about inoculation due to the fact that doctors and apothecaries promoted medication and treatment for their own material gain, regardless of its effectiveness.

Edward Jenner discovered a smallpox vaccination in 1798. He noticed that some milkmaids had lesions on their hands, and determined that cowpox had been transmitted to them by milking cows. He proposed that the cowpox rendered them immune to smallpox. Jenner tested this theory by vaccinating a young boy with material from a milkmaid's lesions, and found it to be true. This vaccination, in comparison to smallpox inoculation, solved

---

50   Kotar, 2013.
51   Ibid.

the issue of smallpox carriers. The vaccine was also a far more reliable defense against smallpox compared to inoculation, and was very unlikely to harm the recipients of the vaccine due to cowpox's mild symptoms. Despite initial opposition, the vaccination was distributed and widely used across Europe by the early 19th century.[52]

Anti-vaccination

Anti-vaccination is not a phenomenon unique to the 21st century; it has been around for thousands of years, and was a particularly strong movement after the introduction of the smallpox vaccine. Discovered in 1798 by Edward Jenner, the smallpox vaccine was criticized by religious groups who claimed it would turn humans into beasts (as the vaccine involved taking lymph from the cowpox blisters of cows).

The vaccination was also initially opposed by many scientists, and other groups simply did not want governments to enforce health regulations. The British government introduced a series of controversial Vaccination Acts beginning in 1840, and lasting until 1898. The first Vaccination Act provided free vaccinations to poor and impoverished citizens who could otherwise not afford to protect themselves from smallpox and may resort to inoculation instead. Inoculation put the uninoculated population at risk of smallpox, and the procedure itself had serious health risks associated with it. The next Vaccination Act in 1853 received more backlash: it made smallpox vaccinations mandatory for all infants during the first three months of life. Parents who refused the vaccination were subject to fines and even imprisonment.[53] In

---

52   Smith & McFadden, 2002.
53   Kotar, 2013.

1867, the government decreed that all children under fourteen years of age must be vaccinated, and introduced laws with cumulative penalties for disobeying. Resistance to the Act was swift and brutal. Violent riots broke out in Ipswich, Henley, Mitford and several other towns. The Anti-vaccination League was founded later that year, focusing on the infringement of personal liberty and choice. The Leicester Demonstration March in 1885 had over 100 000 anti-vaccinationists in attendance and prompted the introduction of the Conscience Clause, which allowed parents opposed to vaccination to receive a certificate of exemption. Anti-vaccination gained significant momentum in the late 19th century United States.[54] Pamphlets and court battles led to the repealing of compulsory vaccination laws in Illinois, California, Indiana, Minnesota, Utah, West Virginia, and Wisconsin, with inspiration for the movement drawn from William Tebb, a well-known British anti-vaccinationist.

Eradication

Smallpox is the only human disease ever to be eradicated. The WHO called for the global eradication of smallpox in 1959, and efforts were intensified in 1966. Eradication of smallpox was possible, as the disease could not be carried by animal hosts, and could only be transmitted between humans.[55] The smallpox vaccination also granted nearly one hundred percent immunity for at least three years, which was very effective in stopping the spread.[56] In 1967, thirty-three countries were endemic with smallpox, and another fourteen reported cases of the disease. A

---

54 Wolfe & Sharp, 2002.
55 Smith & McFadden, 2002.
56 Bremen, Arita, n.d.

mass vaccination initiative was introduced by the WHO around the globe, and surveillance methods were utilized to track outbreaks. Ring vaccination was primarily used, and it involved quarantining infected individuals as well as people who had/would come into close contact with them.[57] This broke the chain of human to human transmission and contained epidemics.

The last smallpox case occurred in 1977 in Somalia, and the disease has been successfully eradicated.

Conclusion

Smallpox was a truly horrific disease that killed millions of people worldwide. Its successful eradication is quite remarkable. While there are concerns that the disease could reappear in an act of bioterrorism,[58] it has presently remained eradicated.

---

57   Ibid.
58   Koplow, 2003.

Chapter 5: 17th Century Great Plagues

Mya Colwell

Introduction

The plague, a disease transmitted largely by fleas infected with the Yersinia pestis bacteria, is a highly infectious disease with a fatality rate of 30-60%.[59] If antibiotics are administered, the fatality rate is considerably lower; however, antibiotics were not available for the majority of the disease's existence. The plague primarily circulates among small animals, and is passed along by fleas who are exposed to the disease once they bite their infected hosts. The disease can be transmitted to humans through a flea bite as well.[60] There have been three pandemics of the plague since the 6th century (two of which were outlined in chapters 3 and 4), and many other epidemics. From 1349 to 1665, there were barely ten years between outbreaks of the disease. The plague caused enormous suffering and drastically reduced populations, while also largely affecting the economy, politics, and social spheres. Population shortages in cities led to an influx of people from the countryside, and the social hierarchy loosened as people scrambled to fill the roles of the deceased. The level of power traditionally held by lower-class individuals rose, in some cases, due to the shortage of workers and the need to keep producing goods. This led to conflict. The plague has not been eradicated, and still exists in areas of Africa, the Americas, and Asia.

---

59   Zietz & Dunkelberg, 2004.

60   WHO, 2005.

Symptoms

As was introduced briefly in previous chapters, the plague appears in three forms: bubonic plague, primary septicaemic plague and primary pneumonic plague.[61] Bubonic plague is the most common form of the disease and it occurs when Yersinia pestis bacteria enters the skin after a flea bite, and travels to the nearest lymph node. Once it arrives, the bacteria replicates at a rapid rate, causing the lymph node to swell painfully. This swollen lymph node is known as a 'bubo', and can occur in any regional lymph node areas along the body (groin, armpit, and neck). Septicaemic plague occurs when Yersinia pestis spreads through the bloodstream, either from direct contact with infected materials through cracks in the skin, or through an infected flea bite. Primary pneumonic plague is less common, but it is the most fatal form of the disease. It usually develops after inhaling aerosolized infected droplets (produced through talking or coughing), and infects the lungs. The plague can then be spread between humans without animal intervention. Symptoms of the disease usually appear three to seven days after the initial exposure, and include shaking, chills, headaches, fever, general weakness, vomiting, and nausea. The disease can result in multiple organ failure, and acute respiratory failure.[62] In primary pneumonic plague, patients often develop a cough and have trouble breathing.

---

61 Ibid.
62 Zietz & Dunkelberg, 2004.

The Plague in 17th century Europe

During the period between 1536 and 1670, an epidemic of the plague broke out approximately every fifteen years, and struck nearly the entirety of Europe.[63] France was hit particularly hard during the first seventy years of the 17th century with approximately two million of its people dying of the disease. 35,000 of these two million died in an outbreak in Lyon in 1629-32. Although Italy is credited with having some of the best preventative measures concerning the plague, they suffered significant losses in the mid 1600s in Rome and Naples. The plague progressed to Germany and the Low Countries, with outbreaks in 1623-24 and 1634-35. Italy suffered outbreaks again in the 1630s, particularly in the central and northern parts of the country. Lombardy, Florence, Modena, and Lucca all had high mortality rates, and a third of the population in Venice is said to have died within the decade. In 1647-50, the plague broke out in Spain, hitting Seville hard in 1649. Half of its population is said to have either died or fled. Between 1647 and 1651, Denmark's population was cut nearly in half, due to plague epidemics and harvest failure. The Great Plague of London in 1665 is a well-known plague outbreak in the 17th century. Meticulous documentation from figures such as Samuel Pepys, a Member of Parliament; Nathaniel Hodges, a prominent physician; and William Boghurst, a respected apothecary, all provide insight into the monumental historic event.[64] The remainder of this chapter will focus on London's Great Plague.

---

63 Porter, 2009.
64 Moote & Moote, 2006.

The Plague enters London

Plague cases first appeared in St. Giles-in-the-fields, a poorer suburb located outside the main London walls, during the winter of 1664.[65] The disease was likely generated internally, as a response to local conditions instead of being introduced through foreign trade.[66] The parish of approximately 1,500 houses continued to be one of the most affected areas until the decline of the plague in October of 1665. Out of the 590 recorded plague deaths in June of 1665, 343 of those occurred in St. Giles.[67]

When the plague broke out in London, the size of the outbreak was initially concealed. This was done primarily to prevent citizens from fleeing the city, as they were needed to keep the economy afloat. As well, accurate death rates would have advertised British weakness to the Dutch in a blazing neon sign. Britain had entered into a war against the Dutch during March of 1665, and they were very concerned about image. These death rates would have also harmed overseas trade. Even when the situation could no longer be ignored, parishes frequently falsified causes of death of their residents, as accurate numbers would have encouraged residents to flee the parish, and would have prevented passersby from frequenting the area. Individual families were also known to bribe 'searchers' to falsify causes of death.[68] If their loved one was officially classified as a victim of the plague, the family home would have been shut up in quarantine for approximately forty days.

Although few cases were initially recorded, the disease began to spread rapidly in the late spring of 1665, and the plague made

---

65 Ibid.
66 Cummins, Kelly, & Grada, 2016.
67 Porter, 2009.
68 Ibid.

its way inside London's city walls during the first week of May. The situation worsened dramatically in June, and by the third week, the death rate was more than twice the normal average.[69] The number of deaths continued to rise over the summer months, and peaked in September with 7,165 Londoners dying in a single week.[70] The disease only began to decline in October of the same year, with the death toll returning to normal in January of 1666. King Charles II and his royal court left London at the beginning of June, with most of London's gentry following suit. As a result, most people with the means to do so fled the city, leaving few physicians to care for the sick, and even less people to dig the graves of the Londoners left behind. Samuel Pepys notes that only a few notable statesmen remained behind including the Duke of Albemarle, the Earl of Clarendon, and Sir Henry Bennet.

Measures taken to slow the spread

The Privy Council started implementing measures to prevent the spread of the disease to unaffected parishes in mid June. These measures were similar to those used during the plague in 1636, and included appointing searchers and watchmen, and building pest houses.[71] Searchers identified houses in which someone had died of the plague, and the local constable was instructed to padlock the door, effectively locking all residents inside, regardless if they were healthy or ill. The door to the home was then marked with a red cross and the words "Lord have mercy upon us", to signify the danger. The house would remain locked for approximately forty days, but this quarantine would be

---

69 Ibid.
70 The National Archives, n.d.
71 Newman, 2012.

extended if another resident died during the initial period. Watchmen were supposed to be stationed outside of infected households to prevent anyone from entering or exiting the home; however, this was not always enforced. Parishes were also responsible for constructing pest-houses. These were buildings where infected people could be taken instead of being quarantined in their homes.

Pest houses were supposed to consist of two buildings: one for those infected with the plague and another for those who appeared healthy, but had been exposed to the disease.[72] Pest-houses were outfitted with nurses and watchmen, and they were encircled with locked gates to prevent the escape of patients. Other precautions taken by the Privy Council included closing theatres, and suspending all school in London from July until September.[73] All public assemblies were forbidden, and taverns, ale-houses, and other entertainment houses were closed. Graves for plague victims were required to be at least six feet deep, and people were not allowed to gather for funerals. To discourage people from attending burials, bodies were buried at night. As the death toll rose, parishes took to digging mass graves which would be filled with fifty or sixty bodies each.[74] Dog and cat catchers were also awarded large sums of money for catching stray animals, as this was thought to prevent the spread of the plague.[75] However, these measures may have been too little too late, as by the end of July, recorded deaths were three times the number recorded at the end of June.

The Great Plague of London was the worst outbreak of the plague since 1348, and approximately fifteen to twenty percent of

---

[72] Ibid.
[73] Porter, 2009.
[74] Moote & Moote, 2006.
[75] Ibid.

London's population perished. The Bills of Mortality listed 68,596 total deaths resulting from the plague, however, experts believe the true number to be over 100,000.[76]

Public Reception

Daniel Defoe's colourful account of the plague year, while largely exaggerated, does reveal public reactions to the plague itself, and the way the situation was handled by government officials. Defoe expresses horror at the number of healthy individuals that were locked in with infected people during quarantine, and this opinion was mirrored by the vast majority of the public. Defoe recounts tales of dramatic escapes from such houses: desperate residents held watchmen at gunpoint, wielded canons, and sent their watchmen on pointless errands only to smash escape-holes in their own walls during his absence. Instances are described where households disappeared mysteriously, seemingly into thin air, leaving their infected residents to die alone. Defoe also remarks that many individuals who did not present symptoms but had been exposed to the disease fled their homes before searchers could arrive. These residents would eventually spread the disease to those who took them in, which was "very cruel and ungrateful". In a brief anecdote, Defoe watches a man cry out in despair as his wife and children are unceremoniously thrown from a dead cart into a mass grave. Although Defoe notes that it would be impractical to neatly lay the bodies in the ground, this passage reveals the callus and perfunctory way death came to be dealt with during the Great Plague. Of the disease itself, Defoe writes that "the swellings, which were generally in the neck or groin, when they

---
76   Zietz & Dunkelberg, 2004.

grew hard and would not break, grew so painful that it was equal to the most exquisite torture; and some, not able to bear the torment, threw themselves out of windows or shot themselves".[77] This bleak description of the disease, and the pain it caused those infected is very evident, and Defoe goes on to claim that those who did not die of the plague could still perish due to the consequences it elicited, namely homelessness, poverty, a lack of a support system, and no means to obtain basic needs.

Treatment and Precautions

London's College of Physicians, England's most elite medical association, typically treated illnesses by balancing the humors: blood, yellow bile, black bile, and phlegm.[78] This was done through a combination of sweating, bleeding, purging, and vomiting. However, Nathaniel Hodges, a prominent member of the London College noted that this approach did not appear to work on patients of the plague.[79] He and other physicians refrained from the bloodletting process entirely, as this seemed to worsen the illness, and endanger the life of the physician further. However, he did advocate opening the pores of patients, and using various liquors to balance the humors. Hodges regularly placed nutmeg in his mouth to ward off the disease, and when visiting patients, he would bring chafing dishes with coals and ignite them in entryways and under beds. He would throw quicklime and herbs on the coals to "destroy the efficacy of the pestilential miasmata".[80]

---

77 Defoe, 2009.
78 Porter, 2009.
79 Moote & Moote, 2006.
80 Ibid.

On an individual level, people protected themselves from the plague with tobacco and strong-smelling herbs, as they believed that the plague was caused by miasmas. William Boghurst, an apothecary, advertised various plague prevention methods including plague water, lozenges, and various drugs that had achieved "wonderful success by God's blessing".[81] Sir Walter Raleigh's cordial was especially popular, and fumigation was encouraged by the Privy Council after a house had been shut up with the plague. People were careful with the food they consumed during this time, as the plague could be transmitted by ingesting plague infected food. Pepys was particularly concerned, as his baker's entire family died of the plague, and his brewer's house was shut up with the disease. Defoe notes that "the Plague defied all medicines; the very physicians were seized with it, with their preservatives in their mouths". One fifth of the college of physicians remained in London during the outbreak, and it is estimated that at least half of these succumbed to the plague.[82]

Conclusion

The Great Plagues of the 17th century brought great suffering, economic upheaval, and tremendous social changes. The Great Plague in London during 1665 was particularly gruesome, and the death of one fifth of London's population will not be easily forgotten.

---

81 Ibid.
82 Ibid.

Chapter 6: Cholera (1817-1923)

Mya Colwell

Cholera: A brief overview

Cholera is a virulent disease that can spread rapidly from region to region and infect large percentages of the population, children and adults alike. The disease spread from the Ganges Delta in India during the early 19th century, and has since caused six pandemics across the globe.[83] Although hundreds of strains of the disease exist, only two, O1 and O139, can become widespread.[84] The seventh cholera pandemic is still currently in effect, and the disease continues to be a public health threat, especially in areas that do not have access to clean water or proper sanitation. According to the WHO, there are 1.3 million to 4.0 million cases of cholera each year, with approximately 21,000 – 143,000 deaths resulting from the disease. The disease can be easily treated with an oral rehydration solution containing sugars and salts, and in more severe cases, patients can be rehydrated intravenously. Eighty percent of patients who receive treatment within an adequate amount of time fully recover, but may need as many as six litres of oral rehydration solution on the first day.[85] These rehydration materials are cheaply obtained and readily available in most areas; however, poor sanitation facilities make it difficult to stop the spread of cholera. In an attempt to prevent senseless deaths, the WHO launched an initiative in 2017 to reduce cholera related deaths by ninety percent before 2030.

---

83 WHO, 2019.
84 Echenberg, 2011.
85 WHO, 2019.

Symptoms

Cholera is an acute diarrhoeal disease caused by the ingestion of the bacterium *Vibrio cholerae*, which can be present in food and water. It can take anywhere between 15 hours and three days until cholera symptoms become evident. Most people do not develop any symptoms of the disease, and those who do usually only experience mild to moderate symptoms.[86] However, the bacteria remains in the faeces of infected patients for one to ten days after the introduction of the disease, and can infect other people once shed back into the environment. The minority of patients who develop severe symptoms of cholera experience excessive vomiting and purging of watery diarrhea. This results in severe dehydration and can kill an infected person in a matter of hours if left untreated.

The First Cholera Pandemic (1817-c.1826)

It is likely that extreme weather conditions resulting from the eruption of Mount Tambora in Indonesia (1815) facilitated the spread of cholera.[87] The eruption caused extreme rainfall and subsequent flooding, which decimated harvests.

The following year was characterized by drought and heat waves, which, although not conducive to the disease, could have compelled people to consume food and water from questionable sources, especially since harvests continued to fail. An extremely virulent cholera outbreak occurred in Calcutta (current day Kolkata) in 1817, and quickly spread throughout the province of Bengal, leaving few towns and villages untouched

---

86 Ibid.
87 Pollitzer, 1954.

by the disease.[88] By 1818 cholera was widespread across India, particularly in Delhi and Bombay (current day Mumbai), and it is estimated that eight percent of the population succumbed to the disease.[89] Technological advancements, colonial expansion, and the economic policies stemming from Europe ensured that cholera could be transported farther than ever before, and in much less time. The disease spread out in all directions, reaching north-easterly into Nepal, Surat, Ceylon (modern day Sri Lanka), Burma (today's Myanmar), Siam (now Thailand), Singapore, and Bombay by 1820, and southernly into the Indian cities of Hyderabad, Bangalore, and Seringapatam. Islands of the Indonesian archipelago and the Philippines were also affected in 1820. Cholera likely reached China in 1817, and Japan in 1822. The disease traveled from Muscat (in Oman) on to the Persian Gulf, parts of Turkey, Iran and Iraq, and even struck parts of Russia. A British military expedition transported cholera from India to Oman in 1821, and the disease quickly spread on to Zanzibar (in Tanzania). The primary recipients of the disease were India, the African coast, Asia, and the Indian Ocean Islands. Cholera spread into the Middle East and the continent of Africa with milder results.[90] Europe and the Americas were spared, for the time being.

The Second Cholera Pandemic (1829-1852)

There is no consensus regarding the origins of the second cholera pandemic. Some historians believe the pandemic sprung out of a recurrence of cholera in Astrakhan (in Russia) in 1830.

---

88   Ibid.
89   Echenberg, 2011.
90   Ibid.

Others cite the Ganges Delta as the origin of the outbreak once again, especially since Bengal had experienced increasingly violent outbreaks in 1826.[91] Warfare, trade, and faster transportation (steamships and trains) made it possible for the disease to spread around the globe in a matter of years. Afghanistan experienced a horrific cholera outbreak in 1829, and from there the disease moved to Persia (current day Iran) and into Russia. From Russia, the disease spread to Bulgaria, advanced through Leningrad (today's Saint Petersburg), and entered Finland, Poland and Austria.

By the June of 1831, Hungary had become infected with cholera, and Vienna succumbed to the disease later in August. Prussia followed soon after. Trade agreements between Prussia (today northern Germany and western Poland) and England made the transmission of cholera to England inevitable, and the disease appeared in London by June 1831. A cholera epidemic occurred in Sunderland on the east coast of England in October later that year. The disease moved on to Newcastle, Edinburgh, and Gateshead. Meanwhile, the death toll steadily rose in London with 97 deaths in November 1831 and 1,519 deaths by March. The total cholera related deaths in 1832 amounted to 5,432 while 14,796 total cases were reported.[92]

Dublin, Ireland was afflicted by cholera in March 1832, and France reported its first cases in Calais in March of the same year. Cholera continued on to Paris, then Belgium, and Norway. The disease made its way into the previously unaffected Portugal and Spain in 1833, and Sweden in 1834. According to historian J.N. Hays, Europe had not experienced this level of panic since the bubonic plague in the 14th century.[93] Cholera had reached the

---

91 Ibid.
92 Pollitzer, 1954.
93 Echenberg, 2011.

distant shores of North America by 1832, through European ships carrying Irish immigrants off the coast of Quebec, Canada. Cholera appeared in the United States in 1832 as well, and had entered Mexico by 1833. The disease spread along rivers, roads, and canals and ravaged Cuba and Nicaragua (1837).

Pilgrims played a large role in transporting cholera in the second pandemic. Cholera broke out among pilgrims in Mecca (in Saudi Arabia) in 1831 and killed, by some estimates, as many as half of them.[94] The entry of cholera into Egypt, Syria, Palestine, and Tunisia is attributed to those traveling pilgrims, returning to their home countries from Mecca. However, compared to the first and third pandemics, these countries were only mildly affected by cholera.

The Third Pandemic (1852-1862)

The third pandemic occurred due to local recurrences of the disease and repeated importations of cholera into infected areas, making it difficult to track the specific spread of the disease.[95] However, we do know that a 1852 outbreak in India caused a violent epidemic of cholera in Persia and Mesopotamia (roughly corresponding to today's Iraq, Kuwait, and parts of Syria and Turkey). By 1853, northern parts of Europe, the USA, Mexico, Canada, Colombia, the northern shore of South America, and the West Indies had been infected with the disease. Greece and Turkey also experienced outbreaks, and the disease was likely brought in by soldiers traveling from the south of France. Cholera spread to Indonesia in 1852, and subsequently to China and Japan in 1854. Cholera spread through the Arabian peninsula into Syria

---

94   Pollitzer, 2011.
95   Ibid.

and Asia Minor, appearing in Egypt and Sudan before entering into Morocco, and the Cape Verde Islands.

The disease also affected previously unaffected areas of Europe including Switzerland, and parts of Austria and Italy. Even Brazil and Venezuela succumbed to cholera, although they had been previously unaffected. A resurgence of cholera occurred in the Philippines in 1858, Korea in 1859, and Bengal later that same year. From Bengal, cholera spread according to its old routes (west in the direction of the Arabian peninsula and Persia, and north-westerly into Russia).[96]

One major advancement that occurred during the third cholera pandemic was the discovery made by Filippo Pacini. He examined the intestines of several cadavers who had died of cholera, and found a large number of curved bacteria inside.[97] However, this knowledge was not widely known, since his discovery was published in a rather obscure journal in 1854, and the relationship between the bacteria and death of the patient was not clearly outlined.

Observations in England also came to light and revealed that contaminated water was a major source of cholera spread.[98] This discovery demonstrated the importance of clean drinking water.

The Fourth Cholera Pandemic (1863-1879)

In the late 19th century, trade routes had changed considerably, a fact that ensured cholera would be spread to new places across the globe.[99] Previous routes led from Persia and

---

96 Barua, 1974.
97 Ibid.
98 Pollitzer, 1954.
99 Barua, 1974.

the Caspian Sea into Europe, but merchants and travelers now passed through the Arabian peninsula, Egypt, and Turkey (Istanbul primarily), to eventually arrive in Southern France and Italy. A large cholera outbreak occurred during a 1865 pilgrimage in Mecca, and it is estimated that 30,000 pilgrims died out of a total 90,000. As the pilgrims returned home on the new trade routes, cholera was able to infiltrate new areas in the Arabian peninsula, Mesopotomia, Syria, Palestine, and Egypt. Alexandria became a center from which travelers and pilgrims spread the disease onwards, through the use of sea routes leading to Mediterranean ports (Istanbul, Marseilles, and Ancona). Cholera then easily spread inland to countries such as Turkey, France, Bulgaria, Romania, Austria, southern Italy, Spain, Portugal, and likely Germany. Italy suffered seriously from cholera, while France, Spain, England and Portugal endured lighter outbreaks. In 1866, after a slight lull, cholera was back in full force. Haeser considers this re-emergence to be "one of the most distressing episodes in the history of epidemics", and this peak was likely helped along by the Austro-Prussian War in 1866.[100] Cholera death tolls ran high, with 90,000 people dying in Russia, 115,000 in Prussia, 80,000 in Bohemia and Moravia (forming today's Czech Republic), 30,000 in Hungary, 20,000 in the Netherlands, 30,000 in Belgium, and 15,000 in England.[101]

The cholera outbreak seemed to die down the following year, but Italy still reported high death rates totaling nearly 113,000. In 1865, cholera devastated Africa, traveling through Aden (south Yemen) across the Red Sea into Somalia and Ethiopia. The region stretching from Kilimanjaro to Lake Tanganyika also became infected, and continued to spread to Zanzibar (70,000 deaths in 1869), Tunisia, Algeria and Morocco.[102]

---

100 Pollitzer, 1974.

101 Barua, 1974.

102 Ibid.

Cholera was present in the United states again in 1865, helped along by awful sanitation conditions in New York particularly.

The Fifth Cholera Pandemic (1881-1896)

When cholera broke out in India and Mecca in the early 1880's, pilgrims, once again, carted the disease all over the world as they returned home. Cholera spread to Egypt, claiming 58,000 lives, and reached Europe, affecting only France, Italy, and Spain.[103] Spain's case fatality was particularly grim, resting at about fifty percent. England and the United States largely escaped cholera outbreaks due to improved sanitation conditions.

However, the disease still ran rampant in South America, affecting Argentina, Chile, Brazil, and Uruguay in the late 1880's and early 1890's. Cholera was also reported in Libya, Tunisia, Algeria, Morocco, Sudan, and Egypt. East of India, cholera was recorded in Indonesia, Sri Lanka, Thailand, Malaysia, China and Japan.

One notable aspect of the fifth pandemic was that Robert Koch conclusively proved that 'comma shaped organisms' cause cholera, due to his studies in Calcutta, and Alexandria. He called these organisms Kommabazillen.[104]

The Sixth Cholera Pandemic (1899-c.1923)

There is no clear source of the sixth cholera pandemic. It could have stemmed from India, or from Egypt or Western Africa,

---

103 Ibid.
104 Ibid.

where cases had not entirely disappeared.[105] In 1900, cholera appeared in Afghanistan and Persia, and during another Mecca pilgrimage in 1902. After yet another outbreak in 1907, Mecca would remain largely free of the disease. Although all efforts were made to quarantine pilgrims returning from infected areas, about 34,000 people died of the disease in Egypt.[106] 1903 saw cases in Syria, Palestine, Mesopotamia, Persia, and Russia. Western Europe reported only sporadic cases of the disease; however, a larger outbreak in Italy claimed 1,400 victims within just a few weeks, and is said to have been brought in by Russian gypsies. Russia was hit hard by the sixth cholera pandemic, with 230,000 cases in 1910.

At the dawn of the first world war, case numbers had dropped slightly in Russia, but continued to ramp up until 1923, with 207,000 cases recorded in 1921.[107] Europe was free from cholera after 1925, but the disease continued to plague China, Manchuria, Japan, Korea, and the Philippines.[108]

Treatment

Cholera treatment during the 19th century tended to do more harm than good. Patients were often encouraged to purge more fluid instead of replenishing lost electrolytes and water levels. Parisian doctors treated the disease by applying a red hot iron to a patient's spine or heel, and other harmful practices involved administering alcohol or morphine to dehydrated patients.[109]

---

105   Pollitzer, 1954.
106   Barua, 1974.
107   Ibid.
108   Pollitzer, 1954.
109   Echenberg, 2011.

European doctors implemented treatment methods from Ayurvedic Indian practices along with treatment consistent with a 'disease of the bile' (according to humoral tradition). They recommended that the cholera patient be given strong liquor, to revive their strength, followed by opium to relax the stomach and bowels. Patients would then be given purgatives such as Epsom salts to rid the body of 'horrid secretions', and they would be prescribed a plain diet as well as a variety of tonics to restore them to full health. Indian doctors prescribed medicine containing ginger, black pepper, aniseed, and borax to purge the body of the disease, and occasionally recommended the usage of opium to dull the pain as well.[110]

Conclusion

Cholera is a horrific disease that has killed millions of people. The fact that the disease can be easily treated makes the death toll even more tragic. It is not medicine that fails patients ill with cholera, but the inability to meet basic needs, such as access to clean water. By improving sanitation and providing reliable methods to purify water, cholera could be prevented entirely.

---

110 Ibid.

Chapter 7: The Third Plague (1855)

Mya Colwell

The plague (a virulent disease caused by the bacterium Yersinia pestis) is known for decimating populations and causing the destruction of entire civilizations. The disease struck fear into the hearts of people for millennia. As stated in chapters three and four, there are three recorded pandemics of the plague, the first being the Plague of Justinian which originated in 542 in the Middle East and the Mediterranean.[111] This pandemic killed millions of people, and chipped away at the Byzantine Empire (eastern Roman Empire), creating an era of instability. The second plague pandemic is known as the Black Death. It originated in 1347 and killed anywhere between one quarter and one half of the populations in Europe and the Middle East by the end of the 14th century.[112] The focus of this chapter will be on the third pandemic, which lasted approximately from 1894 to 1950 and originated in 1855 on the Himalayan border between India and China.[113] Aided by British steamships, the plague soon reached every continent and caused around fifteen million deaths. These deaths were primarily concentrated in India, China, and Indonesia, and the third plague was the first instance, compared to previous plague outbreaks, where the death toll was considerably higher in poorer countries. The third pandemic elicited suffering and fear across the globe.

---

111   Echenberg, 2002.
112   Ibid.
113   Ibid.

Symptoms

The third plague, like the two plague pandemics before it, was caused by the bacterium *Yersinia pestis*. However, the strain of plague present during the third plague was distinct from both the Justinian Plague strain and the strain that caused the Black Death.[114] The disease was likely transmitted by fleas carried on black or brown rats, but some historians are skeptical that rats were major reservoirs of the plague. The plague has an incubation period of about one to seven days after which patients exhibit fever, elevated body temperature, and other symptoms such as chills, head and body aches, weakness, and vomiting.[115] As stated in previous chapters, in bubonic plague, bacteria from a bite of an infected flea travels through the lymphatic system and rapidly replicates once it reaches a lymph node. This causes the lymph node to swell painfully into a 'bubo'. *Y. pestis* bacteria replicate every two hours, and although initial bacteria are ingested by the body's white blood cells, the bacteria soon develop antigens and replicate within these white blood cells. When the disease becomes advanced enough, the inflamed lymph nodes may become open sores accompanied by pus. As the disease progresses, the number of bacteria cells becomes 10 million to 100 billion per gram of tissue, effectively defeating the immune system. In most cases, this results in major organ failure.[116] The plague has a fatality rate of approximately fifty percent, and even healthy people can easily succumb to the disease. Today the disease can be effectively treated with antibiotics, but if left untreated, patients can die within a week after the appearance of a bubo.

---

114 Bramanti, Dean, Wallow, & Stenseth, 2019.

115 WHO, 2017.

116 Echenberg, 2002.

The Spread

The third pandemic originated in 1855, in the Chinese province of Yunnan, and killed nearly two million people there. The plague spread to the southern coast of China and was carried along opium and tin routes by infected rats that nested in opium bales and among other trade items.[117] Soldiers also played a role in transporting the disease. In 1867 the disease had reached the Gulf of Tonkin and spread further on Chinese junks. The plague arrived in Canton and Hong Kong by 1894, and began to cause large epidemics. This marked the official beginning of the third plague. The plague made its way across the globe soon after, reaching Macao in 1895, Formosa (modern Taiwan) in 1896, Bombay (now Mumbai) in 1896, Japan, and the borders of Iran and (present day) Pakistan later that year.[118] The plague spread to the rest of India from Bombay, and went on to affect South America, South Africa, and western North America. In India, it is estimated that 12.5 million people died of the plague between 1898 and 1918, while South America lost about 30,000 people. The disease entered countries through major ports, such as the ones located in Bombay, Singapore, Alexandria, Buenos Aires, Rio de Janeiro, Honolulu, San Francisco and Sydney.[119]

The plague emerged as a threat to Europe in two instances in the late 1800s: during an outbreak of pneumonic plague in Vetlianka, Russia, and when two sailors from Bombay died of the disease while on a ship to London (1896). In the first case, French, British, Austrian, and German governments sent their scientists to study the outbreak in Russia. Unfortunately, instead of making scientific advances, these scientists brought the plague back with

---

117   Echenberg, 2010.
118   Sihn, 2017.
119   Bramanti, Dean, Wallow, & Stenseth, 2019.

them and caused over 400 cases of the disease.[120] The second instance regarding the sailors from Bombay prompted officials, particularly in Venice, to police ships coming from infected areas, and carefully enforce higher levels of hygiene on ships, and among crew members, passengers, and goods.[121] Europe's death toll only totaled about 7,000 people between 1899 and 1950, which was mild compared to the millions of deaths that occurred during the first and second plague pandemics.

Germ Theory

The third pandemic coincided with the beginnings of germ theory. Governments all over the world frantically searched for treatment and ultimately a cure for the plague. In 1894, both the Japanese and French governments sent bacteriologists to study the disease - Shibasaburo Kitasato and Alexandre Yersin, respectively. Both of these men discovered new bacteria in plague patients and found the same bacteria in the organs of rats who had died inside plague infected areas.[122]

Yersin accurately described the characteristics of Yersinia pestis, correctly identifying the bacterium as gram-negative.[123] Kistasato on the other hand, incorrectly identified the bacterium as slightly motile. However, in subsequent years there has been dispute over which individual should be credited with producing the first description of the bacterium.

---

120 Ibid.
121 Ibid.
122 Zietz & Dunkelberg, 2004.
123 Ibid.

Rats and the Plague

A number of scientists, including J. H. Lowry, Alexandre Yersin, and Emile Rocher noticed that rats seemed to be dying in greater quantities inside the borders of plague infected areas, especially in China and India. This suggested that rats were somehow involved in the transmission of the disease. Jean-Paul Simond confirmed this theory in 1898, establishing that while rats could not pass *Y. pestis* on to humans themselves, the fleas who bit infected rats could.[124] The two species of rats present during the third pandemic were the black rat (*Rattus rattus*) and the brown rat (*Rattus norvegicus*). There is still dispute regarding which species of rat contributed most heavily to human cases of plague during the late 19th to mid 20th centuries. Although black rats were better climbers and tended to make nests in walls and ceilings of human dwellings, the species was never present in overly large numbers, especially since the cold European climate prevented the rats from venturing far from buildings.[125] Brown rats were abundant in European cities at the dawn of the 20th century, although they preferred to make their nests in soil or sewage pipes. So, although brown rats had a more sizable population, black rats were able to come into closer contact with humans.

Sanitation authorities began to search for dead rats in their cities, especially on ships coming in from foreign countries. They used early bacteriological methods to test black and brown rats for plague.[126] Results of these bacteriological tests were usually negative, and plague infected rats were only found regularly in East Suffolk, Britain, between 1906 and 1918.[127]

---

[124] Bramanti, Dean, Wallow, & Stenseth, 2019.
[125] Ibid.
[126] Echenberg, 2002.
[127] Bramanti, Dean, Wallow, & Stenseth, 2019.

It is important to note that it is not only the fleas commonly found on rats (*Xenopsylla cheopis*), and other animals such as cats (*Ctenocephalides felis*) that carried the plague; fleas that primarily feasted on human hosts (*Pulex irritans*) could also carry the disease, making it possible to spread the plague without rat carriers.[128] The Third International Congress on School Hygiene in 1910 concluded that one out of three children were infested with vermin (fleas, lice, etc.) and this could have contributed to the spread of the plague. These children usually came from lower socioeconomic backgrounds and tended to live in unsanitary living conditions. Poverty stricken communities, especially, could spread the plague from person to person through the fleas present in clothing, rags, and grain sacks.[129] The fact that the plague could spread without rat intervention makes some historians question the extent rats played in carting the disease through cities and around the world.

Preventative Measures

Although governments were taking steps to prevent the plague, treatment and a cure for the disease remained elusive even at the dawn of the 20th century. Previous beliefs persisted, including the notion that the plague was extremely contagious between humans, and was caused by miasmas. Countries slowly became aware of the link between sanitation and plague rates, and as a result, various sanitation conferences were held. These conferences were held in Venice in 1892, Dresden in 1893, and Paris in 1894. Two of the more notable conferences were the 1897

---

128 Ibid.
129 Ibid.

International Sanitary Conference in Venice, and the conference held in Paris in 1903. These conferences attempted to establish quarantine rules, and introduced new sanitation practices to slow the spread of the plague.[130] They also saw the creation of the Office international d'hygiène publique (OIHP) which would enforce the new rules.[131] This organization would eventually become the WHO. Isolation, incineration, and inoculation were rules implemented by the OIHP, but in most instances, the rules proved to be less than successful. Isolation was essentially quarantine, and entire families of plague victims, and even their neighbours, were shut up in their homes for a period of ten to twenty days, usually under terrible conditions.[132] This not only prompted people to hide their dead, but did little to stop the spread of the disease; pneumonic plague (when the disease infiltrates the respiratory system) was the only instance in which the plague could be transmitted from infected people to their healthy counterparts, and these cases occurred only very rarely. Incineration proved to be slightly more effective than isolation. This was the practice of burning plague infected clothing, bedding, and occasionally entire homes.[133] While this would have killed bacteria and fleas, the fires likely caused potentially infected rats to flee, and carry the plague with them to new areas. This practice would also have caused great distress to people with little means. Inoculation appeared in the form of a vaccine developed by Waldemar Haffkine in 1897; however, it had questionable side effects, and only reduced the risk of infection by about fifty percent.[134]

---

130 Echenberg, 2002.
131 Ibid.
132 Ibid.
133 Ibid.
134 Ibid.

Countries also attempted to curb rat populations once it was made clear that rats were vectors of the disease. Rats were trapped or killed through a variety of poisons, resulting in millions of rodent deaths each year. However, this did little to effectively diminish the rat population, especially since truly effective poisons were expensive, and unobtainable in poorer countries. Western countries likely had more success by rat-proofing their warehouses. After an onslaught of smallpox, yellow fever, and cholera, cities were prompted to improve their hygienic conditions by redesigning sewage systems, providing citizens with a safe and clean water supply, and destroying slums. The introduction of washing machines, vacuum cleaners, and regular baths to European households after 1950 also played a role in decreasing the plague outbreaks.[135]

Antibiotics, specifically streptomycin, were first used to treat the plague in 1945.[136] DDT also became effective at controlling vectors of the disease, but this chemical can be exceedingly harmful to ecosystems, and is banned in many countries today.

Conclusion

The third plague was not as devastating as previous plague outbreaks had been to Europe, but significant death tolls still occurred in India, China, and Indonesia. While the plague only existed in reservoirs in central Asia at the dawn of the third plague, the disease had migrated and established reservoirs in all continents by the mid 20th century.[137] Since the plague emerged from China and Hong Kong, there was significant scapegoating

---

135 Bramanti, Dean, Wallow, & Stenseth, 2019.
136 Echenberg, 2002.
137 Ibid.

and discrimination against Asian communities, blaming them for the onset of the disease.[138] This is not unlike the prejudice and hate directed toward Asian individuals during the COVID-19 pandemic. Plague cases continue to appear today, albeit in smaller numbers. It is estimated that 2,000 cases of the plague occur every year, primarily in Africa, Asia and South America,[139] and eleven countries are currently experiencing outbreaks of the plague. This pandemic was the first of its kind to clearly reveal glaring public health inequalities between wealthy and poor nations.

---

138 Ibid.

139 WHO, 2017.

Chapter 8: Spanish Flu (1918 – 1919)

Sriraam Sivachandran

Background

The Spanish Flu pandemic that started in 1918 is widely considered as one of the deadliest pandemics in history. In scientific terms, the Spanish Flu is a type of Influenza A and to be more specific the subtype is H1N1. This is comparable to the H1N1 swine flu and that is why some people suggest that the Spanish Flu strain originated from the swine flu strain. For patients that were infected the mortality rate was estimated to be more than 2.5 percent. This value was significantly higher compared to the mortality rates of other influenza pandemics and epidemics. Furthermore, the estimated death toll of the Spanish Flu was roughly 50 million.[140] Even though these statistics prove that this pandemic was lethal, it is the uncertainty around these numbers that truly pop out. Considering that the pandemic was first recorded starting in 1918, it would have been hard to collect all the necessary information pertaining to the pandemic, and the modes of information tracking they had back then are miniscule compared to all the resources we have at our hands today. Bearing in mind there are many uncertainties surrounding the Spanish Flu, for it to still be recognised as one of the deadliest pandemics in history speaks to the harm it caused to various populations in the world.

Even though the complete origin of the Spanish Flu is uncertain, there is some important background information that

---
140 Taubenberger, 2006.

can help uncover the mysteries that surround this pandemic. First of all, there is the misconception that this pandemic was named the "Spanish Flu" because it originated in Spain. However, many scientists and researchers have confirmed that the pandemic's origin is actually unknown. The reason that Spain was stigmatized was because the pandemic coincided with World War 1. During the war, the main countries that participated like Germany, the United States, and Great Britain, all shut down their newspapers and even went through the trouble of restricting certain reports. However, as a neutral country, Spain reported the initial facts of the pandemic through their newspapers and reports. Spain did not help their cause when they decided to put out various reports that their king, Alfonso XIII, had contracted the flu. This resulted in the rest of the world assuming that Spain was the epicentre for the pandemic which led to naming the pandemic, the Spanish Flu.[141] The origination and the name of this Spanish Flu is just one of the misconceptions and uncertainties that shows why information surrounding this pandemic needs to be more well researched.

The normal flu-like symptoms that appear in humans usually occur in the fall or winter. However, the Spanish Flu pandemic hit the world in three substantial waves. These waves all occurred in the same twelve-month period between 1918 and 1919. While all the pandemic's waves did not have the same impact, their ability to coincide with each other in only a twelve-month period is what caused great harm to the populations around the world.[142]

---

141 Andrews, 2016.
142 Taubenberger & Morens, 2006.

The First Wave

The first wave of the Spanish Flu hit the world in the Spring of 1918. This wave of the pandemic hit North America, Asia, and Europe in a two-month span. While there are many reports and literature about the Spanish Flu as a whole, it is very difficult to find lengthy reports pertaining to a single wave. However, PBS released an article about how the first wave of the Spanish Flu hit Americans across the United States. For example, many farmers and prisoners had symptoms that aligned with dangerous symptoms of the Spanish Flu. However, due to their lack of knowledge of pandemics, doctors just put it off as the common cold thus resulting in a very nonchalant initial approach of fighting the illness. The first wave of the Spanish Flu showed its true strength during World War 1. During the spring of 1918, a staggering number of American troops were deployed every month in order to combat their enemies in Germany. What they did not know was that the majority of the soldiers were carrying the Spanish Flu, and this even resulted in some soldier's deaths while they were travelling to Germany. Since World War 1 was ongoing, the spread of the Spanish Flu was quite easy and rapid because there were so many people in each countries' army, and they were all fixated in such small quarters. This resulted in the quick transmission of the flu throughout the war and this possibly led to the quick spread of the Spanish flu in Asia and Europe.[143] However, the first wave of the pandemic was not considered deadly. Although there was rapid transmission, the symptoms that patients had were similar to the flu which lead to an also similar mortality rate.[144] Even though the first wave of the Spanish Flu is not highly regarded as the most dangerous wave, it was

---
143 Public Broadcasting Service, n.d.
144 Taubenerger & Morens, 2006.

what started the whole pandemic and that led to the Spanish Flu eventually having more fatalities than World War 1.

The Second Wave

The second wave of the Spanish Flu was at its peak in the Fall of 1918. After the first wave, there was a period of time where there were not many cases popping up around the world. However, once September hit the pandemic started to show its more dangerous effects to various populations. Just like the first wave, the main spread of the Spanish Flu was caused by the constant travelling of various army troops around the world. For instance, one of the main indicators of the second wave of the pandemic was an outbreak that occurred in an army camp located near Boston. Two sailors in the American army contracted the flu and this led to the onset of the second wave of the pandemic. The difference between the first wave and the second wave of the pandemic was the severity of the symptoms that patients exhibited. The symptoms ranged from lack of oxygen to bleeding from noses and ears. Astonishingly, the fear of the pandemic in the United States resulted in many establishments in communities to close down. Since they already felt the effects of the first wave of the Spanish Flu, people specially in the United States started to take many precautions. For instance, people who did not wear masks in public could have been penalised with jail time. Another precaution they took was implementing a staggered approach to different businesses. This was a great idea as it resulted in lower human to human to exposure in the public.[145] Even with these heightened precautions, the increased severity of the Spanish flu during the second wave resulted in

---

[145] Roos, 2020.

the most casualties of any wave. That is why the second wave is classified as the most dangerous wave of the Spanish Flu.

The Third Wave

The third and final wave of the Spanish Flu occurred during the winter of 1918 and the spring of 1919. There is little information about the spread of the Spanish Flu during the third wave, however there are some important timestamps that helped pinpoint when transmission of the flu may have occurred. By the winter of 1918, World War 1 had finally come to an end. That may have suggested that the spread of the Spanish Flu caused by war had finally stopped. However, the Spanish Flu is still transmitted for two simple reasons. First of all, different groups of people celebrated the end of the war. Due to the large number of people in a close environment, the spread of the flu was quite easy. Another reason the flu still spread after the war was because all the soldiers started to go back home. Therefore, if they had contracted the disease at war, there was a high likelihood that they would spread the illness once they went back home. The Spanish Flu also spread quite easily during the third wave because winter is known as peak influenza season. This meant that this was the perfect environment for the transmission for any influenza's strain. However, efforts taken by different countries helped fight against the third wave. For instance, the United States began offering various education programs that helped teach the public of proper etiquette while coughing and sneezing. Municipal governments even gave hospitals money in order to research efficient treatment of this flu strain.[146] However, slowly by slowly the Spanish Flu was eradicated in many states of the

---
146 Centers for Disease Control and Prevention, 2018.

United States and other countries in the world and it was finally eliminated around the whole world by the summer of 1919. The eradication of the Spanish Flu ended what was a miserable but monumental time in human medical history.

Impact

The main reason why the Spanish Flu is considered one of the deadliest pandemics in history is because it affected all age groups with no discrimination. Before the Spanish Flu, other influenza epidemics caused fatalities in the young children age group and the senior age group. The Spanish Flu on the other hand not only affected those specific age groups, it also affected the adult range from twenty years old to forty years old. Even with increased quarantine efforts and education programs during the second and third wave, the lack of knowledge and resources is what led to such a great number of fatalities. Surprisingly, the death rates of people in that specific age range was twenty times higher compared to death rates of previous years. The main cause of the increased fatality rate among young adults can be related back to their childhood. For instance, if someone were exposed to a virus at a young age, they would most likely develop resistance to a virus that has similar characteristics to the original virus. However, if at a young age they are not exposed to any virus or there is an unfamiliar virus, they would most likely not be able to handle the upcoming virus. The second situation is what occurred with the young adults of 1918. At a young age they were not exposed to any dominant strain of the flu and this resulted in a weak response from their immune system when they unfortunately contracted the Spanish Flu.[147] By attacking

---

147 Taubenberger & Morens, 2006.

various age groups, the Spanish Flu left its mark as the deadliest pandemic in recent history.

Conclusion

Uncertainty surrounding anything is inevitable because you can never know anything without hundred percent facts and evidence. The fact that the Spanish Flu originated in 1918 is the biggest hurdle that prevents us from stating definitely the actual origin and final statistics of the disease. However, with the resources we have at our hand today, it is possible to actually try and uncover some of the secrets that surround this pandemic. For example, in 2005 a Center for Disease Control and Prevention (CDC) microbiologist actually synthesized the flu in their lab in order to find out information about the flu that may help with future outbreaks.[148] If the doctors and researchers of 1918 had the resources that we had today, there should be zero doubt that they would have handled the Spanish Flu pandemic at a greater and more efficient rate. They did not have the proper drugs to fight against the early symptoms of the virus. They did not have any idea of the proper synthesis of a vaccine that can actually combat the virus. These are things that they could not control due to the lack of resources in that time period. The major mistake they committed was downplaying the seriousness of the disease and putting first priority into the war. While it may seem easy to judge their decisions hundred years after, there is no excuse for withholding information from the public. Not only does that make the governments look secretive, it causes great amounts of unsettlement throughout the public.

---

148 CDC, 2019.

Even though it is considered the deadliest pandemic due to the staggering statistics, the impact of the Spanish Flu can be truly felt as it introduced a benchmark at how pandemics and virus outbreaks should and should not be handled.

Chapter 9: Asian Flu (1957 – 1958)

Sriraam Sivachandran

Impact and Spread

The Asian Flu pandemic that started in 1957 is another pandemic in our history that had a significant impact on various populations around the world. This influenza pandemic first appeared during the spring of 1957 and lasted until the early months of 1958. It is one of the more popular pandemics that occurred in the 20th century, which includes the Spanish Flu and the 1968 influenza pandemic. However, what made this pandemic different from past pandemics is that the strain of this influenza was different. At this specific time period, this virus type was new and to be specific, the Asian Flu type was Influenza A and the subtype was H2N2. In totality, the number of estimated fatalities worldwide was about 1.1 million.[149] Being forty years in advance of the Spanish Flu, this time around doctors and other healthcare officials were more knowledgeable towards the idea of pandemics and how to identify and handle them if an outbreak did occur. The increase in knowledge led to more capacity for innovative ideas and solutions for a cure. Due to the advancement of technology and the increase in knowledge, the total number of fatalities was undoubtedly lower compared to previous pandemics. However, it is important to note that even though scientific advancements helped produce vaccines, there were still some issues that hindered the response to the pandemic. The good news of a quick vaccine response should not masquerade the fact that the government still could not put out an efficient

---
149 Centers for Disease Control and Prevention, 2019.

response for all cities to follow.

Unlike the Spanish Flu of 1918, there is no uncertainty around why the Asian Flu got its name. This influenza pandemic is also known as the Asian Flu due to its origin. The Centers for Disease Control and Prevention reported that the Asian Flu was first officially reported in Eastern Asia, specifically in February 1957 in Singapore. The significance of the name is correctly portrayed as the pandemic quickly spread throughout Eastern Asia. For instance, in April of 1957, thousands of inhabitants of Hong Kong reported feeling the effects of the Asian Flu. Not only was this the first significant outbreak of the Asian Flu, but this was also the onset of other eastern Asian countries contracting the Asian Flu. For example, in May, the pandemic spread to the eastern Asian country of Taiwan and over hundred thousand Taiwanese citizens contracted the virus. From there, the timeline of the Asian Flu continued to India, where in the month of June over one million citizens contracted the virus. However, the true strengths of the virus showed itself in the month of August. While there were some isolated cases of the Asian flu in the United States of America and the United Kingdom in the months of June and July, it was not until August when there was a serious outbreak. It is important to look at how the Asian Flu spread in the United States and the United Kingdom because these were two of the western countries that were significantly affected by the Asian Flu. In the United States, there were many minor outbreaks that occurred over the summer of 1957. Many of the outbreaks took place in western coastal cities as these cities were closer to the continent of Asia. By the conclusion of the pandemic, over 116,000 estimated United States citizens died due to the pandemic. On the other hand, the British Journal of General Practice provided many details on how the Asian Flu affected the United Kingdom. Throughout the month of September, many countries a part of the United Kingdom started recording many cases of the Asian Flu. These countries included Wales, England, and Scotland. By the end of December, there were an estimated 3550 deaths between both England and Wales. Between the months of January and March of 1958, there were numerous cases and deaths of the Asian Flu in the United States and the United Kingdom.[150] The significance of these cases was that the majority of the affected patients were actually senior citizens. After these last outbreaks, the number of cases and deaths of Asian Flu had died down and this ultimately led to the eradication of the Asian Flu.

Symptoms

Like any virus, there were a number of symptoms that patients may have exhibited if they contracted the Asian Flu. However, the type and severity of the symptoms varied for various age ranges. The Asian Flu attacked people in two and three phases. The second phase was the harshest as it lasted from two to a maximum of fourteen days. The unique phenomena surrounding the Asian Flu was that patients showed the symptoms in a similar pattern. Initially, they would be feeling minor effects of vertigo such as instability in the lower body area and they would be feeling body chills, which led to extreme weakness. Many of the symptoms were similar to regular influenza virus. For instance, Asian Flu patients exhibited runny nose, sore throats, and high fever. Fortunately, compared to the Spanish Flu, the majority of the patients only had these minor symptoms. Specifically, out of all the Asian Flu cases, there were only complications in 3% of those cases. Some of the more major symptoms included pneumonia, bronchitis, and specific cardiovascular diseases.

---
150 Jackson, 2009.

Many seniors were susceptible to the virus as their weak immune systems were no match for the virus and this unfortunately led to death. However, it was children and young adults that had the highest infection rates. This was because both of these age ranges were able to come in contact with many people. For instance, the virus spread throughout the children population because they still went to school during the pandemic. On the other hand, the virus spread steadily in the adult population because amenities such as public transit was the ideal place for the virus to spread to a large mass of people.[151]

Response

When the Spanish Flu occurred in 1917, the scientific knowledge surrounding pandemics and epidemics was quite minute. Due to the lack of knowledge, it took a longer time to identify the problem and figure out a solution. As the years went by, more people started to get educated on all pandemics and they started to understand the severity surrounding the effects of the pandemic. Different countries had different initial responses. For instance, in Great Britain different doctors had different initial approaches to combat the virus. For example, one doctor decided to prescribe antibiotics to patients that did not exhibit any severe symptoms. An example of one of these antibiotics was penicillin. On the other hand, there were some doctors that thought the antibiotics were better suited for patients that showed severe symptoms.[152] However, there was some previous knowledge on different experimental vaccines that were developed in the 1940s and 1950s that helped isolate a cure. For instance, in 1952 the

---

151 Jackson, 2009.
152 Jackson, 2009.

World Health Organization was able to create certain vaccines that helped with regular seasonal influenza cases. Unfortunately, since this virus was a different strain compared to previous influenza viruses, there was no time for certain countries to react properly.[153] For instance, when the Asian Flu hit the United States hard in September, they were completely prepared compared to when the virus initially hit Hong Kong. United States healthcare officials were able to create a virus which eventually helped save millions of people's lives around the world. The Centers for Disease Control and prevention utilised different healthcare companies in order to create the vaccines just in time. An estimated 5.4 million doses of the vaccine was released, and the majority of those vaccines were for the population while some of the doses were given to the United States Defense Department.[154] That is one of the reasons why compared to the Spanish Flu, the total number of fatalities of the Asian Flu was quite low.

Even though there were many advancements in the scientific community, there was still the fact that certain non-scientific problems arose during the pandemic. Since the United States is a distinguished and first world country, there are many documented reports on how they reacted to the news of the pandemic. Even though they did have a quick response by creating the vaccines, they did not use proper procedure to help sustain the health of all their citizens. Doctors throughout the United States could not agree on the severity of the virus. Some doctors thought the virus was mild and it was not necessary to take the vaccine. There was plenty of evidence that shows that there was disorganization and a lack of communication between healthcare officials and the citizens. Firstly, one of the areas where the United States faltered is regarding children. Like it is today, school started in the fall for all students. Unfortunately, the fall was when the United

---

153   Barberis et al., 2016.

154   Brown, 2009.

States was hit the hardest. Even after hearing that the virus was spreading quickly throughout the United States, some people in certain communities thought the virus was a hoax so they decided that school would continue. It was clear that this was the wrong response as many children contracted the virus and this led to many children not attending school and the infected children had eventually transmitted the virus to their respective families. They finally decided that it was important to propose a staggered response to the reopening of businesses. There is similarity between the approach taken in regard to the Asian Flu and how the Ontario Government responded to the Coronavirus pandemic. The provincial government was late regarding the closure of schools and they also proposed a staggered approach to the reopening of business using the three different phases. Another problem with the United States' response was how they controlled their borders. For example, there was a boat of exchange students coming from the Netherlands to the United States. Some students were banned from going on the trip as they contracted the virus. However, by the time the boat arrived in the United States, approximately 29% of the students on board contracted the virus.[155] The border control problem seen in 1957 is different from the strict border control laws that are in place today. If there were stricter laws pertaining to border control back then, more people would have been saved.

It is very peculiar how even in 2020, the response to the pandemic was just as slow and disorganized as the response to the Asian Flu. It is concerning that governments still have not learned how to respond properly to pandemic and epidemic situations that arise in their country. Even if there is an economic deficit, governments need to realise that their citizens' health should be the first priority. However, it is unnecessary to completely forgo all the positive things that the healthcare

---

[155] Little, 2020.

officials and government did in response to the news of the pandemic. It is easy to forget that the pandemic occurred in 1957 and back then they did not have quite as much resources as we have today. Nevertheless, they were able to create vaccines using recent research and they were able to finally eradicate the Asian Flu in approximately one year. The scientific progress that was seen in healthcare officials that responded to the Asian Flu was evident when compared to the Spanish Flu. This progress was important to see because it showed people around the world that as the years go by, even if viruses mutate, there will always be responses that change in response to the present situation.

Chapter 10: Swine Flu (2009 – 2010)

Sriraam Sivachandran

Background

One of the most recent pandemics that caused havoc around the world was the 2009 swine flu. Surprisingly, there was not a single pandemic in the forty years leading up to the swine flu of 2009. This strain of the swine flu had a small resemblance to the 1917 Spanish flu, as they both were a type of Influenza A, and the subtype for both pandemics was H1N1. The reason that this influenza virus was so unique was because it made doctors and healthcare officials deal with new information. They had never come into contact with this type of virus compared to the other H1N1 viruses that were documented. The first human case was reported in April of 2009 and the World Health Organization finally concluded that the pandemic was eradicated in August of 2010. Due to inaccuracies throughout various reports, the Centers for Disease Control and Prevention estimated that the number of fatalities around the world ranged between 151,700 and 575,400 in just the first year. Furthermore, they also estimated that the mortality rate was between 0.001% and 0.007% for the swine flu, which was actually quite low compared to the mortality rate of the Spanish flu.[156] Within the first four months of the pandemic, the World Health Organization identified the continents with the most cases and deaths. They reported that North America and South America had the most cases and deaths while Africa

---

156 Centers for Disease Control and Prevention, 2019.

had the least. Fortunately, compared to past pandemics, the resources available for doctors and other healthcare officials was readily available as there was more information pertaining to pandemics and technology around the world had seriously augmented. Due to these advantages, various antiviral drugs and vaccines were produced in order to fight the swine flu. Even though the 2009 swine flu resulted in many fatalities, it is commendable how healthcare officials learned from past pandemics and reacted as quickly as possible to eradicate the pandemic.

Before the 2009 swine flu pandemic infected humans around the world, it is important to understand that the swine flu is not actually known for infecting humans. The swine flu is actually an influenza virus that affects pigs and results in respiratory problems. The swine flu that appeared in 2009 surprisingly only affected humans and did not affect pigs. Due to increased technology, references, and reporting, specific information, and dates of the timeline of the swine flu had been recorded. According to the Centers for Disease Control and Prevention (CDC), the first case of the swine flu had emerged on April 15 in a ten-year-old that resided in California. After just two days on April 17, an eight-year-old was also infected in California. As soon as the two novel cases of the swine flu were reported, the CDC started working on an eligible vaccine. Unfortunately, the swine flu started to spread all across the United States. The months of May and June were when the number of cases and hospitalizations of the swine flu really amplified in the United States. For example, by the end of June all fifty states of the United States had cases of the swine flu. There were an initial thirty countries with cases of the swine flu and after the first serious wave, there were an estimated 213 countries that had been affected by the swine flu. The first wave of the swine flu occurred throughout the spring and early summer of 2009 while the second wave hit the world in late November with a decline in the number of cases occurring in July.[157] Due to the fact that healthcare officials were exposed to more useful reporting tactics and efficient technology in 2009, the origin and spread was documented thoroughly, and all useful and relevant information became accessible.

Symptoms

Some of the symptoms that are exhibited by patients of the swine flu are similar to the seasonal influenza virus. Generally, the swine flu affects one's upper respiratory tract and, in some cases, it affects the lower respiratory tract. An incubation period of a disease represents the amount of time it takes for symptoms of the disease to go away, starting from the first day the symptoms were actually present. The average incubation period of the swine flu is two days. On the other hand, the contagious period is the amount of time a patient of a disease can give the disease to other people. If a person were infected with the swine flu, they could start infecting other people as soon as one day or as long as a week after becoming infected. However, if this patient had a weak and under-developed immune system, they would be able to infect people for a longer period of time because it would take longer for them to stop exhibiting symptoms.[158] Symptoms such as chills, coughs, and sore throat are prevalent in swine flu patients.[159] Many other symptoms of the swine flu are similar to symptoms of other strains of influenza. These symptoms are the ones that last the shortest amount of time as they are not quite as serious. Furthermore,

---

157 Centers for Disease Control and Prevention, 2019.
158 Jilani et al., 2020.
159 Mayo Clinic, 2019.

if a person is healthy and has a strong immune system, the symptoms would not last as long and they will not be too serious. Unfortunately, there are always complications that arise with several symptoms of any disease. If complications occur and patients require hospitalization, then there is no doubt the virus would prolong its existence. If a patient has pre-existing lung related diseases, they are susceptible to some dangerous complications such as pneumonia, bronchitis, and in some serious cases, death. If a patient does not handle the initial symptoms well, then there is a possibility that they would feel the effects of some of the more serious symptoms and this could happen if the patient does not handle the symptoms in the first two days of their incubation period. Healthcare officials identified certain risk factors that if present in patients may result in death. Based on various reports, healthcare officials were able to identify which age ranges and types of people were easily susceptible to the swine flu. First and foremost, people with pre-existing health problems were easily susceptible to the virus because they had weakened immune systems and this included citizen of all ages. Another age range that was easily susceptible to the swine flu were children who were younger than five-years old. Since they were just born, their immune system was not developed enough, and it did not have enough experience to fight against the virus. Lastly, pregnant women were susceptible to the swine flu because carrying the fetus results in the body having a harder time to defend against the virus. For instance, some of these risks' factors include lung diseases and obesity.[160] Even though some of the symptoms of the swine flu are similar to other strains of influenza, that did not stop the swine flu from causing many fatalities.

---

160 Jilani et al., 2020.

Treatment

For any disease or virus, there are multiple treatment methods that may decrease the effects the symptoms have on a patient and this is the case with the 2009 swine flu. The type of treatment that a patient receives depends on how severe their symptoms are. For example, patients with non-severe symptoms usually just stayed at home in order to rest. They would have battled their symptoms by being hydrated and utilising antibiotics. On the other hand, the situation and circumstances are completely different for patients exhibiting severe symptoms. For instance, doctors recommend that these specific patients should immediately visit the hospital and they should be admitted in the intensive care unit. There are also specific antiviral drugs that can help decrease the effects of the symptoms. The antiviral medications used to treat the swine flu are oseltamivir, zanamivir, and peramivir.[161] All of these medications positively affect the genetic makeup of the swine influenza strain and this leads to the decrease of symptoms. However, by the month of July, healthcare officials in three different countries found out that a specific strain of the swine flu was resistant to oseltamivir. There were also vaccines that were eventually developed to help battle and prevent the swine flu. By April 21st, the CDC already started working on the development of a novel vaccine that could help deal with the initial symptoms of the swine flu. However, by the month of October, the official swine flu vaccine was given to citizens of the United States. Finally, in the month of December over hundred million doses of the official swine flu vaccine were available, and any citizen was able to get the vaccination if they wanted to.[162]

---

[161] Jilani et al., 2020.
[162] Centers for Disease Control and Prevention, 2019.

Response

Many governments around the world had similar responses on how to deal with the 2009 swine flu. This was facilitated with help from global health organizations like the World Health Organization and the Centers for Disease Control and Prevention. One of the key early responses provided by the government and these organizations was how the swine flu spread among humans. They were able to identify that the virus spread throughout humans using airborne particles and these particles were able to sit on objects and can be spread to other people if they come in contact with those specific objects. The CDC also executed the plan of using field teams in various countries in order to collect data and inform healthcare officials of the proper protocol. A monumental response to the 2009 swine flu was when the World Health Organization officially declared the virus as a pandemic. Slowly, the CDC worked with several governments and healthcare organizations in order to monitor all the cases around the world. Overall, by the end of the pandemic the CDC was able to estimate the total number of cases, deaths, and hospitalizations using all the data they collected.8 Considering all the progress that the scientific community had made from past pandemics, the response for the swine flu pandemic was quite efficient.

Even though the swine flu pandemic caused havoc across the world, it is important to note that humans have learned from their past. It is impossible to limit human to human contact and therefore it is inevitable to completely limit an enormous increase in the number of cases. However, the efficient and quick responses that various governments and organizations put in place helped ease the public's distress. Despite the fact the pandemic lasted a year and half, the various surveillance systems and data collection teams had done enough thorough work in order to put in successful treatment and eradication plans.

Chapter 11: Ebola Virus (2014 – 2016)

Sriraam Sivachandran

Before the coronavirus pandemic of 2020, the most recent global pandemic that plagued the world was the Ebola virus, which first appeared in 2014 and lasted two years, until 2016. There have been minor outbreaks that occurred in the past, but the 2014 outbreak was by far the biggest Ebola virus ever. Like other diseases, there are various strains of the Ebola virus that have different characteristics. In the case of the 2014 outbreak, the strain was the Zaire Ebola virus species. The significance of this Ebola outbreak was that the first case appeared in a village in the western African country of Guinea. Furthermore, it was not until August 8th of 2014 when the World Health Organization listed the western African outbreak as an international concern. In the early stages of the outbreak, the virus spread to certain western Africa countries such as Mali, Senegal, and Nigeria. However, there was also minor international spread of the initial Ebola virus outbreak as the virus spread to Spain, Italy, the United Kingdom, and the United States. The World Health Organization considered the 2014 Ebola outbreak eradicated on March 29th, 2016. After the eradication of the Ebola virus, the Centers for Disease Control and Eradication estimated the total number of cases and deaths that occurred throughout the pandemic. They reported that Sierra Leone had the most total cases while Liberia had the most total deaths. On the other hand, they reported that countries outside of Western Africa that had cases of the Ebola virus did not have that many cases and deaths. For example, Spain, Italy, and the United Kingdom all had only one case and all those countries reported zero deaths. The United States reportedly only had eleven cases of the Ebola virus and fortunately there was only one confirmed death. In total, there were 28,616 people that had contracted the virus and 11,310 had died from the Ebola virus. Based on all the final estimates of total cases and deaths, various healthcare organizations understood that this outbreak hit the countries in western Africa the hardest.[163] One would think that in 2014, the increase in scientific and medical knowledge throughout the years should have helped the various healthcare organizations around the world to rapidly eradicate the virus. However, some important factors that played a major role were environmental factors and cultural factors. Due to these circumstances, the effects of the outbreak were prolonged until 2016.

How did it start?

The first ever known outbreak of the Ebola virus occurred in Africa in 1976. Surprisingly, there were two outbreaks that occurred at the same time in two different African countries: The Democratic Republic of Congo and Sudan. The reason Ebola Virus got its name was because the outbreak that occurred in the Democratic Republic of Congo was relatively close to the Ebola river. Pertaining to the 2014 Ebola outbreak, evidence of the first case of the Ebola virus was seen when a one and half year-old boy was exhibiting serious symptoms of previous Ebola cases. The toddler resided in a small village in the country of Guinea. Unfortunately, he started showing symptoms that were very similar to previous Ebola cases and he died due to the severe symptoms. The toddler's family had also died from Ebola

---

163 Centers for Disease Control and Prevention, 2009.

symptoms as they contracted the virus from the boy. After that, there were five reported cases of Ebola in the same village and this was a result of the fast transmission of the virus. The virus then spread to the capital city of Guinea, Conakry. After the quick spread of the virus in Guinea, the virus had spread rapidly to a couple of other western African countries, Sierra Leone, and Liberia. Western Africa was the main origin of the Ebola virus and this area was unfortunately plagued with the most cases and deaths. Unlike other past pandemics, there was not that much international spread of the virus from the actual origin point of the virus. In September of 2014, a man flew back home to Dallas, Texas from a country in western Africa and was reported to have Ebola-like symptoms. Unfortunately, he succumbed to his symptoms one month later. Even though the patient was in the hospital, before he died, he transmitted the virus to the two doctors that were treating him, but fortunately they recovered properly from the virus. Another United States citizen infected with the virus was identified in October of 2014. This person was a healthcare worker who volunteered in Guinea. He was a patient in New York City that fortunately recovered. The Center for Disease Control and Prevention reported that most of the international cases that were identified were a result of people who volunteered in the western African countries as healthcare workers. For example, there were seven people that had contracted the virus and out of the seven, six patients survived. Slowly but surely, the number of cases of the virus in the western African countries increased to a point where Guinea, Liberia, and Sierra Leone had double the amount of cases and deaths compared to neighbouring countries. After about one and a half years, the first western African country to initially be eradicated of the Ebola virus was Liberia. This occurred in May of 2015. However, healthcare officials reported minor cases of the Ebola virus over the summer of 2015. The pattern of reporting no cases one month and having Ebola virus another month lasted until the next year in June 2016. Liberia was deemed Ebola virus free in March of 2016 while Guinea was deemed Ebola Virus free in June of 2016.[164]

Contraction and Transmission

The area where the Ebola virus and other famous pandemic viruses differ is the actual transmission of the disease. A person can contract the virus if they come in contact with certain animals. For instance, if someone gets in contact with certain organs and bodily fluids of animals there is a great chance, they may contract the virus. The animals that could transmit the virus are bats, monkeys, and chimpanzees. In the case of the 2014 Ebola outbreak, it was reported that the first patient of the Ebola virus contracted the virus from a fruit bat, but it was not known which bodily fluids the patient got in contact with. After contraction from animals, a patient of the Ebola virus can transmit the virus through simple human to human direct contact transmission. There are two ways that the virus can be transmitted between humans. The first way the virus can spread is by directing healthy people to blood and bodily fluids of infected or dead patients. A person can also contract the disease if certain objects they touched were contaminated with infected bodily fluids. In the case of the 2014 outbreak, a major disadvantage that caused hectic setbacks was the fact that the outbreak occurred in west Africa. The setback was that the countries of western Africa were developing countries. Due to this fact, it was not possible to contain the disease at a quick pace. An important fact to note was that several healthcare

---

[164] Ibid.

workers that were volunteering in the western African countries contracted the disease. Unfortunately, because of the bad healthcare situations, the healthcare workers worked in improper stations while treating patients and this led to them easily contracting the disease. Another reason that the virus spread so quickly throughout the western African countries was the culture in those countries. For example, when the villages wanted to bury the dead patients, they did not adhere to proper rules and regulations and this led to direct contact with dead bodies. The World Health Organization gave specific advice to villages to use trained burial teams to bury their loved ones in order to limit the human to human transmission. Another set of people that was easily susceptible were the family members of people that were infected. It may be considered obvious that these family members are easily susceptible but in the case of the 2014 Ebola outbreak it is important to factor in. This was because in the western African countries, families had no choice to stay in their homes even if there was an infected person situated at home. Those families were not as fortunate as developed countries' families, and this ultimately led to the rest of the family being infected. Considering that the western African countries were severely underdeveloped compared to other countries, it was no surprise that the outbreak spread so quickly throughout those countries.[165]

Symptoms

The signs and symptoms of the 2014 Ebola virus outbreak were fairly similar to past Ebola virus outbreaks. For instance, if a person were to contract the virus, the time it would take for

---
165 World Health Organization, 2020.

the person to actually start exhibiting symptoms ranged from two to twenty-one days. The onset of symptoms occurs in two phases, with the first phase resulting in patients exhibiting fairly common symptoms to other viruses. For example, some of the first symptoms to appear were fevers, fatigue, and headaches. Patients also initially felt muscle pain and sore throat, but there was no guarantee which initial symptoms would appear first because many of the symptoms would appear unexpectedly. While the initial symptoms of the Ebola virus were not that serious and dangerous, the second phase of symptoms to appear were definitely more serious and caused more damage. Patients were reported to experience vomiting, diarrhea, and moderately damaged kidney and liver function.[166]

Treatment

There were certain treatment options that healthcare workers used in order to eliminate certain symptoms because there was no one ideal treatment method that healthcare officials recommended. One of the most popular treatment methods was rehydrating the patient with intravenous fluids. This may seem like a simple treatment method, but it was effective in cases outside of the western African countries. One of the main reasons that the western African countries had the most cases and deaths was because they did not have the resources to help cure the virus in their patients. In 2015, an experimental vaccine was proposed to combat the Ebola virus and it was quite successful. Specifically, there were 5837 people that decided to use the vaccine and it was reported that no person had contracted the virus after ten days. Based on background

---

166 Ibid.

information of the Ebola virus, there are certain prevention methods that anyone can take into consideration. People that are susceptible to the virus should limit direct contact to infected animals and infected humans in order to avoid contracting the disease. If there is an outbreak, healthcare officials should do their due diligence in a rapid manner in order to contain the outbreak as fast as they can, so the virus does not spread to other communities.[167]

Due to the fact that the 2020 coronavirus has caused havoc throughout the world, it seems like the 2014 Ebola outbreak occurred a very long time ago. Surprisingly, unlike the coronavirus, the 2014 Ebola outbreak did not spread rapidly to international countries outside of the western African countries. The glaring message that can be learned from the 2014 Ebola outbreak is the discrepancy in the healthcare situations in third world countries. This is the main reason why the virus spread so quickly in Guinea, Liberia, and Sierra Leone. Even though international healthcare volunteers decided to come to those countries to help nurse patients, there was a great chance that they also contracted the disease. If these western African countries had the healthcare technologies and establishments that developed countries had, there is no doubt that the 2014 Ebola outbreak would have been contained at a more efficient rate.

---

167 Ibid.

Chapter 12: COVID-19

Michael Tang

An overview of COVID-19

The current global COVID-19 pandemic began in late December, 2019, in the city of Wuhan in the Hubei province of China. Evidence suggests that the outbreak began at the Huanan Seafood Wholesale Market in Wuhan, meaning that the virus was likely transmitted to humans from animals.[168] Initially, there was a cluster of 41 patients with pneumonia of an unknown cause, with many of the cases connected to the seafood market. It was later discovered through lab testing that the cause was a new type of coronavirus. Coronaviruses are a group of viruses that contain large single-stranded RNA and can infect humans and animals. The disease caused by the new coronavirus was named "COVID-19" by the WHO on February 11th, 2020.[169] For the purposes of this book, the coronavirus itself will also be referred to as COVID-19.

The elderly, people with preexisting conditions and healthcare and essential workers are the most at risk groups to COVID-19. The elderly are especially at risk due to their weakened immune systems. Next, people with respiratory conditions may be unable to take safety measures such as wearing a mask. Finally, healthcare workers and other essential workers would have the highest potential exposure to COVID-19 compared to other groups in the population. Patients with more severe cases of COVID-19 may require a ventilator, a machine that can help a patient breathe or breathe for the patient.

---

168 Zhai et al., 2020.
169 Secon, Woodward & Mosher, 2020.

Symptoms

The initial symptoms of COVID-19 include coughing, fever and other respiratory symptoms.[170] More severe complications such as pneumonia can develop as a result of COVID-19. However, not everyone who contracts COVID-19 develops symptoms. This is known as being "asymptomatic". This is one of the reasons why COVID-19 can be hard to contain, as some people infected with COVID-19 may unknowingly spread the virus and/or may not follow proper infection control measures due to a false sense of security.

The virus can be spread through direct contact or through respiratory droplets produced during actions such as speaking or coughing. There is growing evidence from numerous scientific studies that COVID-19 can be spread through microdroplet production, which means that the virus can be spread through airborne transmission at a distance greater than the two meters in social distancing guidelines.[171] This is another major reason why COVID-19 has caused such a large-scale global pandemic.

International response

China's first response was to close down the Huanan Seafood Wholesale Market on January 1st, 2020. The city of Wuhan was then placed under quarantine on January 23rd. From January to February, cases begin to appear, and case counts begin to grow in other countries such as South Korea, Iran, the United States and Italy. Italy was hit particularly hard by the virus, forcing the government to place all 60 million of its residents under

---

170   Zhai et al., 2020.
171   Ahmed, 2020.

lockdown on March 8th. The WHO declared the COVID-19 outbreak a pandemic on March 8th as case numbers grow across the world.

On March 13th, US President Donald Trump declared a national emergency.[172] He then decided to suspend $400 million in funding for the WHO on April 14th as he felt that the WHO did not adequately respond to the COVID-19 pandemic. This is a devastating blow to the international agency as the US is the WHO's largest donor.

Many countries around the world have implemented travel bans or restrictions and infection control measures such as lockdowns and quarantines to prevent the spread of the virus. These have been accompanied by economic restrictions or shutdowns. Non-essential businesses, such as restaurants and salons were ordered to close until further notice. These restrictions were eased as the rate of cases decreased. In general, countries that were less severely affected by COVID-19 imposed stricter lockdown and infection control policies.

The attitude that the national government takes towards COVID-19 largely determines how much the country is affected by the virus. Two examples of this principle are the US and Brazil, two countries that have not managed to control the spread of COVID-19 as of July 2020. These two governments have both downplayed the severity of COVID-19 at times and have rushed to reopen their economies at a faster rate than health officials recommend.

The American government has at times been too focused on reopening the economy at the cost of unsustainable increases in infection rates and deaths. Infection control policies such as social distancing and the temporary suspension of non-essential business do have the effect of hurting a country's economy. However, it is crucial to not rush the reopening of the economy, as noted by Dr. Anthony Fauci, the leading infectious diseases and

---

[172] Secon, Woodward & Mosher, 2020.

coronavirus expert in the US.[173]

As such, Trump and his allies have been at odds with infectious diseases experts at times due to their desire to reopen their economy as soon as possible without much consideration for public health. It is likely that the Trump administration wants to get the American economy back to normal as soon as possible for Trump's re-election bid in November. Recently, Dr. Fauci has said that his media appearances have been limited by the Trump administration as he advocates against the reopening of the US economy at the moment. The aggressive reopening policies taken by the US government has contributed to the rising case counts in the US and the inability to control the spread of COVID-19.

On the other hand, government officials in Brazil, the second hardest-hit country (as of July 2020), did and still do not take the virus seriously even after President Jair Bolsonaro himself was infected with COVID-19. President Jair Bolsonaro had repeatedly downplayed the severity of the virus and likely got infected after refusing to follow social distancing guidelines himself.[174] Some cities and states in Brazil have also reopened earlier than health officials had recommended, further contributing to the spread of COVID-19.

The role of the WHO during the pandemic

The WHO was created in 1948 to facilitate international health efforts. Its role is especially important during a pandemic of a global scale. The WHO can warn countries around the world of health emergencies, like when it declared a global health

---

173   Reuters, 2020.
174   Reuters, 2020.

emergency on January 30th 2020[175] in response to increasing infection rates across the world. During COVID-19, the WHO has mainly focused on forming committees to determine advisories and other recommendations on how to respond to the virus.

The WHO has been criticized before for having slow responses to emergencies due to a preference to wait for scientific consensus before acting.[176] For a pandemic like COVID-19, time is of essence due to the infectious capabilities of the virus. The WHO has also come under fire recently from the US government and scientists over its handling of the pandemic. Some members of the US government believe that WHO was heavily influenced by China and that the agency did not properly handle the current crisis. US president Donald Trump decided to withdraw the US from the WHO on July 7th, 2020. The president had said in White House announcements that Chinese officials withheld information from the WHO and that the WHO was pressured to publish "misleading" information.[177]

The WHO also resisted calls by scientists to acknowledge that COVID-19 can be spread in the form of micro droplets. The WHO had maintained that the virus is spread through sneezing and coughing and that a social distance of two meters was enough to prevent the spread of the virus. However, COVID-19 spreading in the form of microdroplets would mean that the virus can spread at distances greater than two meters. The WHO has recently changed its stance on how COVID-19 is transmitted by acknowledging that the virus can be transmitted through other actions such as talking. Overall, although the WHO will need to make some reforms after its post-pandemic review, the agency is still important in global health situations such as pandemics.

---

175   Velavan & Meyer, 2020.

176   Weaver, 2020.

177   Weaver, 2020.

Infection control

At this point in time, there are no reliable cures or treatments for COVID-19. Thus, infection control and prevention are especially important right now. The main methods of infection control that have been recommended for everyone are as follows: social/physical distancing, using masks and other PPE (personal protective equipment), handwashing and disinfecting frequently touched surfaces. The combined effect of everyone following proper infection control guidelines can really help to slow down or contain a pandemic.

Social distancing mainly involves staying at least 2 metres away from other people and avoiding public places and gatherings.[178] This is to minimize direct and close contact with others, which is how COVID-19 spreads. However, it may be more accurate and beneficial to use the term "physical" distancing instead as "social" distancing suggests that a person must socially isolate from friends and family. A person can still socialize without physical contact via phone, social media, email etc. Avoiding direct, physical contact does not mean that you must also socially isolate yourself. Keeping in contact with family and friends also helps to maintain positive mental health and reduce stress.

The use of masks and other PPE are essential in preventing a person from both spreading and being infected with COVID-19.[179] These can also include face shields, gloves and barriers (like you would see in a grocery store). The most important type of PPE is the face mask, and it is the form of PPE that is the most recommended and is even being enforced by law in some countries. Masks can prevent an infected person from

---

178 Public Health Agency of Canada, 2020.
179 CDC, 2020.

spreading COVID-19 through airborne transmission, and this is especially important as some people may be asymptomatic spreaders of COVID-19. It is important to note that pre-packaged masks are only usable for one day at most. Reusable masks can be purchased or self-made, but they must be washed daily.[180]

The other forms of PPE (masks, gloves, etc.) can be helpful in infection control but are not the most effective forms of PPE. For example, face masks cannot fully prevent a person from spreading the virus through airborne droplets. Face masks are more useful for protecting the eyes. Next, gloves can be useful during activities such as grocery shopping. However, it is important to note that gloves are not a substitute for proper hand washing and sanitizing.

Handwashing is also important as it prevents a person from transferring germs and viruses to an entry point such as the mouth and the eyes.[181] We often use our hands while eating and it is common for people to touch their faces with their hands. Handwashing is especially important after being in a public place and touching surfaces such as doorknobs. When hand washing is not possible, a hand sanitizer should be used.

Cleaning and disinfecting are especially important for frequently touched surfaces such as doorknobs, desks and chairs.[182] This is important as germs and viruses can remain on surfaces in an active form for a period of time. Cleaning should be done before disinfecting, and it involves the removal of impurities using soap and water. Disinfecting involves the use of disinfecting sprays, wipes and other products. This helps to further kill any remaining germs and viruses left over on the surfaces.

---

180 CDC, 2020.
181 Ibid.
182 Ibid.

Potential treatments and vaccines for COVID-19

Potential vaccines and drugs that can treat COVID-19 are currently undergoing testing and review. Some of the more promising treatment options at the moment include: antiviral agents, chloroquine and hydroxychloroquine, corticosteroids and convalescent plasma transfusion.[183]

As COVID-19 is caused by a virus, some form of an antiviral drug should theoretically be able to treat COVID-19. The use of pre-existing antivirals such as remdesivir are currently being tested. Next, chloroquine and hydroxychloroquine (a very similar drug to chloroquine) are antimalarial and anti-viral drugs that are also being tested. Corticosteroids could also be useful in preventing inflammation in the lungs. Finally, convalescent plasma transfusion refers to the transfer of plasma from patients who have recovered from a disease to patients who currently have that disease. Plasma is the liquid component of human blood, and convalescent plasma refers to the plasma of a patient who has recovered from a disease. The aim is to use a plasma transfer to transfer immunity to a disease from one person to another.

However, until reliable treatments and vaccines are developed and fully tested, we can only try to control the spread of the virus through the infection control policies and practices mentioned earlier in this chapter.

---

183 Zhai et al., 2020.

Chapter 13: Future Pandemics

Michael Tang

Preventing and fighting pandemics in the future

COVID-19 will not be the last pandemic that humanity will experience. There will always be infectious diseases present in our world, and it is up to us to either learn from our mistakes or repeat them. There are many actions that we can take to try to limit the severity of pandemics in the future or perhaps prevent them altogether. We can try to reduce our exposure to pathogens and improve our responses to those pathogens. Some of the major directions we can take include reducing wildlife trade and habitat exploitation, investing more in virology research and public healthcare systems and adapting cutting-edge technology such as AI into our pandemic responses.

The largest source of human diseases: Wildlife

Zoonotic diseases refer to diseases that spread from animals to humans. Around 60% of known human disease and 75% of new emerging diseases are zoonotic in nature.[184] Indeed, the current COVID-19 pandemic started at the Huanan seafood market where live animals were being sold, and bats are believed to be the original source of this zoonotic disease. Other notable examples of zoonotic diseases include Ebola, Zika virus and SARS. Millions of people die every year from zoonotic diseases, especially in poorer countries.

---

[184] Bhalla, 2020.

The prevalence of zoonotic diseases in our world is largely due to 7 trends: the rising demand for animal protein, mass exploitation of natural resources and urbanization, the wildlife trade, intensive agriculture, food supply changes, increased travel and trade and climate change.[185] Our intensified exploitation of the natural world has simultaneously increased our exposure to natural pathogens. Global travel has increased the rate of which a disease can spread across the world. Climate change has also changed the habitats and behaviours of some animals that may be carriers of zoonotic diseases. We must develop strategies for sustainable agricultural and developmental practices to avoid overexploiting habitats and creating zoonotic diseases. Protecting the natural environment would also be beneficial for biodiversity and for fighting climate change in addition to reducing the prevalence of zoonotic diseases.

Investing in research and databases

Next, it is important to note the importance of investing money in research to stop a pandemic. Historically, poorer countries were affected to a greater extent during a pandemic due to deficiencies in healthcare and infrastructure. A more coordinated flow of money during a pandemic would certainly help poorer countries respond to internal issues. Private businesses were also hit hard by the economic shutdowns during the pandemic. Businesses can prepare for pandemics by doing risk-assessments, creating pandemic mitigation plans and getting pandemic insurance.[186] If there is even insurance for terrorism attacks, then why is there not insurance for pandemics?

---

185 Ibid.
186 Wolfe, 2020.

Another potential action we can take is to invest more resources in studying viruses and enhancing the study of virology. The Global Virome Project is a proposed project that will create an inventory or database of viruses in animal populations with the potential to infect humans.[187] This project would cost billions of dollars but would have an impact similar to that of the Human Genome Project. The Human Genome Project revolutionized medicine as mapping human DNA contributed to our understanding of the human body and the treatment of genetic disorders. Overall, creating a human virome (a database of all viruses that can infect or reside in humans) is a very important investment to make if we want to combat viral diseases in the future.

We can also set aside some of the money currently being allocated to combat COVID-19 into a fund to prepare for future pandemics. This money should be mainly invested into three areas: diagnostics, drugs and vaccines.[188] This is so that we can better test for, treat and vaccinate against the next pandemic-causing disease. The current COVID-19 virus is a relative of SARS, a coronavirus that caused a pandemic in the early 2000's. Large amounts of money were spent funding investigators during the pandemic, but funding dropped off after the dust settled. Continued research on coronaviruses after SARS could have helped with our current COVID-19 situation. Short-termism is indeed a problem when it comes to research, and we must continually invest in virus and disease research even when we are not experiencing a pandemic.

Unfortunately, it is hard for us to continually invest time and resources to combat issues that only take effect in the future. These include issues such as preparing for future pandemics

---

187 Ibid.
188 Mui, 2020.

and climate change. While these are major issues, they lack pressing concern and are not really considered in our short-term plans. While we can't really do anything to change our natural fixation on the short-term, we need to collectively address this by setting aside resources right now to prepare for future issues. For example, we could take 2% of the trillions of dollars we are spending on combating COVID-19 and invest the money into coronavirus, virology and vaccine research. Overall, we must create plans for these long-term problems and continually invest time and resources bit by bit towards solving these issues.

Improving healthcare systems

Improving our healthcare systems is an obvious step forward. Public health systems must be able to respond to a pandemic in a coordinated and scientifically driven fashion. Countries that effectively responded to COVID-19 (such as Taiwan and South Korea) all had solid healthcare infrastructure, a coordinated response and provided trustworthy information to their citizens.[189] The major components of their responses focused on the deployment of massive human and technological resources to provide testing and contact tracing. Countries such as the US did not respond well to the virus due to factors such as disorganization, a lack of scientific-based decision-making and a lack of funding for local and state healthcare units. The attitudes that some governments had taken towards COVID-19 as a whole and mask usage should be addressed to ensure that all countries will effectively respond to a future pandemic.

---

189 Lu, 2020.

Hospitals can also be better designed to handle outbreaks. One possible modification could be to use an ambulance bay area to screen patients before they enter the hospital. This area could then be cut off from the rest of a hospital if an incoming patient is suspected to be infected with an infectious disease. Negative pressure zones could also be installed and used in an emergency to limit the spread of airborne pathogens.[190] Another possible modification could be to design rooms that can quickly be converted into a critical care ICU room. Finally, hospitals and clinics could also install systems that allow healthcare providers to contact and treat patients remotely, which would reduce direct contact between patients and healthcare providers.

Improving infrastructure and urban design

Besides improving research and health infrastructure, we can also redesign our cities, buildings and transportation systems to be able to respond more effectively to a pandemic. Urban design can have a huge impact as we become increasingly urbanized and densely populated and because we spend most of our time indoors every day. We could design public spaces so that they can also function as logistics and treatment areas in an emergency.[191]

Airports could add more security screening lanes and/or incorporate automated screening lanes to reduce congestion and person-to-person contact.[192] Screening could also be done before passengers get to the airport, such as on the shuttle buses heading to the airport. Overall, we need to improve airport

---

190 Peters, 2020.
191 Ibid.
192 Peters, 2020.

screening procedures and design as travel is one of the main ways a disease can spread across the world.

In the modern world, people spend most of their time indoors. As such, improving air quality and installing screening processes and sensors in our buildings could have a large impact. Increasing the flow of fresh air would reduce a person's exposure to pathogens in an indoor setting. We could use newer forms of air treatment systems such as using UV light air cleaners.[193] Sensors that can detect the presence of viruses and other pathogens in real time could also be installed. These sensors could then trigger an alarm and/or activate air cleaners. Another possibility would be to screen people as they enter a building. Temperature checks can be used to detect fevers and affected people would then be directed to a treatment centre or into self-quarantine to avoid infecting other people.

We can also redesign our neighbourhoods to promote general health as common conditions such as high blood pressure can make someone more susceptible to a disease like COVID-19.[194] This could involve building more green spaces, parks and improving walkability. Walkability refers to the degree to which a neighbourhood promotes walking as a method of transportation and recreation. Walkability can be improved by building more sidewalks and improving the aesthetics of a neighbourhood (e.g. building more parks). Exercise and increased sunlight exposure (a good source of vitamin D) has been linked to a lower risk for conditions such as high blood pressure. Building more green spaces would encourage outdoor activity and improve air quality. This is important as air quality is better outdoors compared to indoors and because polluted air has been linked to a higher

---

193 Ibid.
194 Ibid.

risk for conditions such as asthma. Improving everyone's general health would reduce the burden on our healthcare system and make our population less susceptible to a pandemic in general.

The importance of handwashing cannot be stressed enough. We can be exposed to various pathogens through commonly-touched surfaces such as doorknobs and elevator buttons. The problem is that there are not many handwashing stations or public washrooms available to ensure that everyone can regularly wash their hands. Handwashing stations or hand sanitizing stations would be especially useful in public places such as public transit stops. Placing these stations in public areas could also reinforce their usage through peer pressure and other people setting an example. Encouraging proper hand hygiene would have a large impact during a pandemic and for combating diseases in general.

Taking advantage of technology

Technology has revolutionized our lives, making it more convenient and expanding the limits of what we can do on a daily basis. We can make use of more technology to improve our response to a pandemic through improving predictions, facilitating global communication and collaboration and providing better platforms for research. One example is creating a digital immunity passport system.[195] Assuming privacy and confidentiality concerns are properly addressed, lab results and other evidence of immunity could be stored digitally and the data could help health officials in planning their next moves and keeping track of who is safe to return to work. Overall, we could definitely take

---

195 Wolfe, 2020.

advantage of the digital world to keep track of health data and better coordinate our response to pandemic.

AI and machine learning are some of the most exciting and promising new technologies being developed right now. AI could be used to analyze molecular, epidemiologic, ecological and climate data to identify areas of the world that are the risk of getting diseases from wildlife. This can allow us to take preventative measures to stop a pandemic from starting in the first place. We can also use AI to detect early signs of an outbreak so that we can respond to a potential pandemic faster. One example is the Global Public Health Intelligence Network is an AI-based surveillance system created by Health Canada and the WHO.[196] This system can analyze more than 20,000 online news articles per day across nine languages, and it was credited for creating the first alerts for SARS and MERS. Pre-existing AI systems that can analyze wildlife and outbreak data need to be updated and built up to a global scale to be useful in the future.

Another potential technology we can use is 3-D printing.[197] This would involve creating blueprints for equipment that could be used to mass produce said equipment whenever they are needed. For example, we could create 3-D printing blueprints for ventilators instead of stockpiling large amounts of the equipment. We could cheaply store hundreds of blueprints for equipment and then choose the right equipment to produce depending on the situation. This technology can also be used in conjunction with standard manufacturing practices to produce larger supplies of vital equipment such as masks and ventilators.

---

196   Lu, 2020.
197   Mui, 2020.

Chapter 14: The Evolution of Pandemics

Michael Tang

The evolution of pandemics

Disease-causing pathogens have always been present in our world and will continue to exist for the foreseeable future. The increase in the human population over time has unfortunately increased the risk of pandemics occurring. As the worldwide population grew, villages and towns became cities. This meant that our population density (how concentrated people are in one area) also grew, which would lead to more close contact and an increased risk of a disease spreading.[198] However, some aspects of how a pandemic plays out have stayed constant while other aspects have changed. Aspects that have stayed constant include stigmatization and an initial phase of ignorance and denial when an outbreak begins.[199] Some of the major changes that occurred in human history that have changed our vulnerability to pandemics include: population growth, urbanization, agriculture, globalization, warfare, the wildlife trade, habitat exploitation, infrastructure development, and technological developments.

---

[198] Walsh, 2020.
[199] Jones, 2020.

Recurring patterns in most pandemics

There are recurring patterns in the course of almost every major pandemic as some aspects of human nature and culture have remained constant throughout history. These patterns mainly involve the societal effects of a pandemic. For example, pandemics have always caused prejudice, from anti-Semitism during the medieval plagues to COVID-19-related anti-Chinese sentiment.[200] Whenever something goes wrong, we always try to find the person or thing responsible. Unfortunately, this tendency can lead to stigmatization and prejudice, especially if a pandemic originated in a single country where the majority of citizens are of a single ethnic group. The uncertainty and stress caused by a pandemic could also have the effect of amplifying pre-existing prejudices as well.

Another recurring pattern is how there is always an initial state of denial when the first outbreak of a pandemic occurs. In the case of the COVID-19 pandemic, the initial response in China was arguably slow and government officials may have tried to suppress early concerns about an outbreak.[201] This is similar to what was proposed by Charles Rosenberg, an American historian who theorized a three-stage structure for a pandemic.[202] The first stage is denial, when people tend to ignore the early signs of an outbreak in order to preserve economic interests and provide self-reassurance. The second stage is recognition, when people search for explanations. The third stage is when the public responds to the outbreak. This pattern has stayed more or less constant throughout history.

---

200 Ibid.
201 Ibid.
202 Jones, 2020.

Agriculture, the wildlife trade and habitat exploitation

Around 12,000 years ago, humans transitioned from a nomadic hunting lifestyle to an agricultural lifestyle. They began settling down in stable locations and began cultivating crops and domesticating animals. This greatly increased direct contact between humans and animals and facilitated the transfer of microorganisms from animals to humans. Some of these microorganisms would have immediately caused diseases, but some of the others would have remained in the human population and eventually evolved into a pathogen.

Human activities that have increased the prevalence of zoonotic diseases include live animal markets, agricultural intensification and habitat exploitation. Running the wildlife trade in populous regions can lead to disastrous consequences such as the H5N1 "bird flu" and the current COVID-19 pandemic, which started at a live animal market in Wuhan, China.[203] Next, the exploitation of natural habitats and resources has increased as agriculture intensifies in order to feed our growing population. When we explore and use new pieces of land for agricultural purposes, we also encounter new wildlife and microbes that could potentially become pathogens. It is an unfortunate consequence of the growing demand for food and resources worldwide as our population continues to grow.

---

203 Morens et al., 2020.

Trade, travel and exploration

Once a pathogen enters the human population, humans become the ultimate spreaders of those pathogens. The main methods through which an infectious disease can spread across the world are through exploration, trade routes and travel. Advances in transportation technology allowed people from across the world to come into close contact and has nullified any geographic barriers a disease could have encountered in the natural world.

The age of exploration or the discovery age was a period between the 15th and 17th known for intense overseas exploration by European powers. While this period has undoubtedly created the connected world we know today, they have also contributed to spread microbes and pathogens across the world. One famous example is how Columbus' voyages to North America caused the "Columbian Exchange", which refers to the exchange of material goods, crops and culture between Europe and the Americas. However, diseases were also exchanged, such as how smallpox was brought to North America while syphilis was brought back to Europe.[204]

Around the year 1320, the Black Death spread to Europe from Asia via major trade routes. The United States experienced several outbreaks of the "American plague" (otherwise known as yellow fever) between 1793 and 1798.[205] It is believed that the disease was brought over by Carribean trading ships. The exchange of commercial goods has always provided opportunities for different organisms to spread across the world, from invasive species to microscopic pathogens.

---

204 Morens et al., 2020.
205 Ibid.

Even before the microbial concept of disease existed, diseases were noted to spread at the same speed as human travel. The 1831 cholera outbreak was followed closely by the media in real time, and it was found that the disease advanced as fast as human travel routes from India to Europe would allow.[206] The development of affordable travel and expanded trade networks have no doubt increased the rate and potential of diseases spreading worldwide. Influenza pandemics have historically been noted to follow human movement and more recent pandemics have followed rail, ship and air routes. HIV is believed to have emerged at some time between 1880 and 1920, but only became a pandemic in 1981 due to increases in the global population and developments in travel and trade networks.

Warfare and conquest

In the past, warfare was a common way that diseases spread across from civilization to civilization. The first recorded pandemic in history occurred in Athens during the Peloponnesian War in around 430 B.C. This pandemic was likely caused when the Spartans laid siege to the city of Athens, causing a massive outbreak within Athenian walls. Warfare is similar to travel and trade in that soldiers essentially "travel" to other parts of the world and can spread any diseases that they are carrying. The soldiers often stay in the areas that they conquered before returning home. Thus, the soldiers spread the diseases that they are carrying in the places that they fight in and can then pick up new diseases and spread those diseases when they return home. A more recent example of this concept is the 1918 Spanish flu. The timing of this pandemic coincided with the end of World

---

206 Ibid.

War I, when soldiers returned home after fighting in Europe. This pandemic killed 50 million people worldwide and 700,000 in the US, demonstrating how warfare can spread diseases across the world.[207] In the 21st century, warfare is not a significant pathway for disease transmission compared to other pathways such as travel and trade due to our world being relatively more peaceful. However, diseases can still be spread during smaller scale conflicts and peacekeeping missions when soldiers return home.

Developments in medicine, public health

A pandemic will continue its course until it has affected all susceptible people or is stopped by societal action. Therefore, medical knowledge and technology as well as public health systems play a large part in determining how deadly a pandemic is. Technology can help us to track and predict outbreaks, allowing us to respond in a timely fashion. Developments in medicine have improved our ability to treat diseases and save the lives of more patients. We have developed vaccines, discovered antibiotics and have improved our knowledge in areas such as virology and anatomy. However, public health policies are far more important during the early stages of a pandemic as the drugs and vaccines needed have not been developed or are not available in large quantities.[208] The initial response by governments and health organizations play a large role in determining the severity and direction that a pandemic will take.

Public health responses to pandemics have also developed over time. The plague pandemic of the 1340's brought about the first quarantines. The "plague tractates" were guidelines for self-

---
207 Lubrano, 2020.
208 Morens et al., 2020.

isolation described in Boccaccio's Decameron.[209] These guidelines encouraged young citizens to shelter away in the Florentine countryside to avoid the plague in large cities. Nowadays, health guidelines during the COVID-19 pandemic include social distancing, the closing or restricting of parts of the economy, limits on gatherings and travel restrictions.

It is important to note that public health policies can range from optional to mandatory policies. Whether or not these policies are enforced can have a huge impact on the course of a pandemic and on societal trust towards their healthcare systems and government. For example, China utilized a public health police to enforce quarantines and restrict movement during the early stages of the COVID-19 pandemic, and it has worked to an extent.[210] Other countries that have managed COVID-19 relatively well, such as South Korea, used aggressive health policies such as mass testing, contact tracing and mandatory isolations. However, there needs to be a balance between informative and coercive health policies. Using less authoritative methods is more ideal for gaining and keeping the public's trust, which will be useful even after the pandemic is over. In general, health policies will gradually become less coercive as the situation improves.

Developments in research, technology and infrastructure

Overall, developments in fields such as pathology and epidemiology and technological advances have improved our ability to track and predict the movement of diseases. Research has contributed to our increased understanding of how a

---

209 Ibid.
210 Ibid.

pandemic plays out and has allowed us to develop treatments for various diseases. However, much remains to be done in terms of research, as evidenced by our current struggles with COVID-19.

Next, technological advancements have made it easier to store and share information, which is important when fighting a pandemic of a global scale. Databases of diseases and viruses have been created, and pandemic prediction systems have been improved with the help of AI. The development of social media and the internet has increased access to information, but at the risk of overwhelming the public with too much information and the potential of misinformation being spread.[211] This can lead to anxiety and confusion as there are many conflicting sources of information and it can be difficult to determine the credibility of a source.

Pandemics have usually spurred the development and redesigning of urban infrastructure and design. Infrastructure such as water sanitation and sewage systems are important in preventing the introduction and spread of diseases in a community. Many diseases and pandemics had a larger impact on less developed countries due to issues such as overcrowding, underdeveloped sanitation systems and underdeveloped healthcare systems. The cholera pandemics in the 1800's led to improvements in sewage infrastructure and the creation of zoning laws to prevent overcrowding.[212] These improvements were necessary as cholera primarily spread through contaminated water.

The current COVID-19 pandemic has also raised further questions about how urban design can accommodate the need for social distancing and other disease control methods. Some potential directions to take could include adding more

---

211 Morens et al., 2020.
212 Peters, 2020.

mini-markets, designing maze-like parks and making cities more compact.[213] Groceries are an essential part of our lives, but with small markets shut down the only options are large supermarkets where social distancing can be hard to maintain. Mini-markets could be set up in public spaces as an alternative to supermarkets. Next, green spaces such as parks could be designed to increase distancing between users. One possible design could be a maze of hedges with sufficiently wide paths to allow for social distancing. Finally, cities could be designed to be more compact, which means that important amenities and services are easily accessible all around the city. This would increase access to medical and health-related services as well as reduce pollution from transportation. Air pollution has been linked to conditions such as asthma, which could make people more vulnerable to an infectious disease.

---

213 Davies, 2020.

Conclusion

Michael Tang

The impact of pandemics

The word "pandemic" comes from the Greek word "pan" (all) and "demos" (people), illustrating a pandemic's widespread impact. As Charles Rosenberg puts it, "Epidemics start at a moment in time, proceed on a stage limited in space and duration, follow a plot line of increasing revelatory tension, move to a crisis of individual and collective character, then drift toward closure."[214] This is indeed a more or less accurate description of an epidemic or a pandemic. Pandemics start with a small outbreak, spread across the world for a limited period, cause individual and societal dilemmas and eventually die out. So far, we have covered 13 of the largest pandemics that have occurred throughout human history. Many of the pandemics were caused by a combination of factors such as warfare, zoonotic spillover, travel and trade and had a huge impact on societal, medical and technological development. As the saying goes, "necessity is the mother of innovation". Past pandemics have spurred us to develop new technology and public health policies. They have forced us to be more wary of the natural world and made us redesign our urban areas and infrastructure. We have overcome them in the past and we will continue to do so using the lessons we learned from the past.

However, it is important that we do not let exaggerated fears of another pandemic change our priorities and/or make us ignore other threats that are already in front of us. There have been

---
214 Jones, 2020.

cases where there was a widespread panic about a pandemic that never materialized. Some examples include fears of Ebola spreading to the US in 2014 and the H1N1 influenza panic in 1976, 2006 and 2009.[215] We need to keep in mind that pandemics occur only when outbreaks get out of control. Proper, scientifically driven prevention and infection control measures can prevent an outbreak from ever becoming a pandemic.

While it is impossible to fully eliminate the possibility of a pandemic occurring, we can greatly reduce the prevalence and impact of pandemics by addressing the risk factors that cause them and by improving the way that we respond to this threat. Pandemics are directly caused by other global issues, with the main issues being a rising demand for animal protein, mass exploitation of natural resources and urbanization, the wildlife trade, intensive agriculture, food supply changes, increased travel and trade, warfare and climate change. The best way to prevent another pandemic is to minimize our exposure to zoonotic diseases by curbing activities such as habitat exploitation and the wildlife trade and by reducing the spread of diseases through trade and travel. If an outbreak does occur, we can recognize the threat earlier through the use of AI and other detection systems. We can then implement quarantines and lockdowns earlier and restrict travel earlier to avoid having the outbreak spread across the world. It may well be impossible to react quickly enough to contain every single outbreak, but we can use all of the experience and lessons learned from past pandemics to improve our response to future threats. It is interesting that all of the global issues listed above are already on our to-do lists. It may in fact be a better idea to indirectly address the threat of pandemics by investing resources into other issues such as combating climate change. Overall, focusing on other global issues at hand

---

215   Ibid.

would have a positive impact beyond reducing the frequency of pandemics and smaller outbreaks.

Potential next steps

We must also remember that other health conditions and activities such as smoking have accounted for an equal or greater number of deaths compared to a pandemic. High blood pressure, obesity and other common conditions can make people more vulnerable to other diseases and health conditions. Smoking kills approximately 7 million people every year and is the leading cause of preventable death.[216] Another example would be how around 5000 people have died in China due to ischemic heart disease during the COVID-19 pandemic[217] (as of April 2020) compared to around 4600 reported deaths due to COVID-19 (as of August 2020).[218] In addition, these common health conditions are often risk factors for infectious diseases such as COVID-19. Improving the general health of our population would decrease the susceptibility of our population to any infectious diseases that we cannot fully control and contain. Overall, while pandemics are a major issue that we need to address, we must carefully weigh the severity of every issue we face and allocate our resources accordingly.

It is important to note that pandemics are more of a societal issue rather than an individual issue. In other words, the combined actions of all members of society will determine whether a pandemic is swiftly curbed or whether it will drag on. This means that the public's trust in science and their

---

[216] CDC, 2020.
[217] Jones, 2020.
[218] Johns Hopkins University, 2020.

government plays a huge role in determining the severity of a pandemic. On that note, a major issue that still needs to be addressed is the general anti-science and anti-government movement. Some notable subgroups of these movements include the anti-vaccine movement, the anti-masking movement and the anti-lockdown movement protesting partial shutdowns of the economy and restrictions on daily activities. After all, a working COVID-19 vaccine would be useless if people refused to take it. People who aren't wearing masks are at a greater risk of getting infected with COVID-19 and spreading it, with the presence of asymptomatic cases making it worse. While vaccines and masks may not seem to have much in common, both groups desire personal freedom over all else and have a fundamental distrust towards the government, health officials and scientists. An example would be how Hugs over Masks (a Canadian anti-masking group) has partnered with Vaccine Choice Canada (a prominent Canadian anti-vaccine group).[219] Scientifically driven policies such as vaccinations are beneficial enough to be enforced, but the problem is that enforcing these policies could cause unrest and help the anti-government and anti-science movement. It is difficult to find a balance between informative and coercive health policies, with the use of coercive policies generally increasing as a pandemic grows worse.

The general premise of the aforementioned movements is the concept of "personal freedom", or that people should have control over any medical procedures done to them and that the government should not tell them what to do. The problem here is that most if not all recommended or enforced health guidelines or interventions exist to protect everyone, not just the individual person. An example of where it would be fine to exercise personal freedom would be a wisdom teeth surgery or orthodontic

---

219 Ireland, 2020.

treatment, as it would just affect the patient. On the other hand, getting vaccinated or wearing PPE protects everyone around you in addition to yourself. We have to remember that we live in a society, not in an isolated world by ourselves. Infectious diseases rapidly spread because humans live together in proximity, whether it be in cities, towns or villages. There are times where one must accept the advice and policies of public health authorities, who are always thinking about the health of the entire society that they are responsible for. Herd immunity occurs when a sufficiently large enough portion of a population is immune to a disease, which makes it harder for that disease to spread. This collective immunity can fall apart if a large enough portion of that population is not immune to the disease or does not take appropriate action.

The age of information and technology has allowed for wide-ranging communication and education. However, it is a double-edged sword in that misinformation can also be widely spread, whether it be unintentional or intentional. The internet and social media platforms such as Facebook can be used to easily spread fake and misleading information. Anti-vaccine groups are often very active on social media, where they use "alarmist" claims to attract attention, such as claiming that wearing masks harm children. They may also spread conspiracy theories, with some examples being that vaccines are part of a larger conspiracy by the government and pharmaceutical industry and that COVID-19 is a scam that the government is using to impose contact tracing to monitor our movements.[220] They may also cherry-pick data and studies by only drawing their information from a select few studies that may or may not be outdated.

However, not everyone is actively trying to access all the information that is available to them. People who have firmly

---

220 Ibid.

taken a stance or side will usually ignore all the information coming from their opposing viewpoints. People who are undecided or sitting on the fence are likely the ones actively looking for information. Thus, it is important for public health officials to deliver clear and reliable information to those who are undecided before they pick a side. Once a person has fully embraced a side or opinion, it becomes difficult to change their minds. An example of an undecided group is the portion of society that is "vaccine-hesitant", or those who are unsure of whether vaccines are safe and necessary.[221] These people will either have their minds changed by public health officials or the anti-vaccine group or will remain undecided. Both the "vaccine-hesitant" and anti-vaccine groups are unlikely to get vaccinated, so it is vital that public health agencies and scientists increase their social media and internet presence.

One potential solution to this has been the rise of scientific journalism and scientific celebrities. There are masters and postgraduate degrees in this field available from universities across the world such as Imperial College London and New York University.[222] These programs prepare young scientists to engage the public and become influential spokespeople of the science community. This is necessary as many scientists simply publish articles and reports of their research in various scientific journals, depending on the authority as a scientist to reach people. However, in the modern world mainstream media and entertainment receive the most attention. On that note, science needs more media icons and celebrities to improve the accessibility of scientific information to the general public. In other words, science needs spokespeople who are as much an entertainer or reporter as they are a scientist. After all, the

---

221 Ireland, 2020.
222 Hotez, 2020.

average person would most likely spend more time checking the New York Times and watching "The Big Bang Theory" than they would spend reading the New England Journal of Medicine. William Sanford Nye (an American television presenter commonly known as "Bill Nye the Science Guy"), Bob McDonald (a Canadian scientific journalist who hosts a weekly radio show called "Quirks and Quarks") and Neil deGrasse Tyson (an American astrophysicist who regularly appears on TV shows and has a YouTube channel called "StarTalk") are good examples of scientific icons. Scientists must adapt their outreach strategies to accommodate the modern world. Producing scientific information through entertainment and the media is one way to go about this. Indeed, we may very well need more science celebrities in the future as people are more likely to listen to a scientific celebrity that they adore rather than a plain scientist telling them what they can or cannot do.

A final message

There is no doubt that pandemics can cause massive disruptions in everyone's daily life. From the threat of the disease itself to restrictions on activities and events, life during a pandemic is stressful and frustrating. It can be difficult to resist the urge to return to normal daily activities, but we must wait until public health authorities determine that it is safe to do so. This will likely mean waiting for a viable vaccine to be widely available and the subsequent development of herd immunity. Trying to return to normal too quickly can give people false hope and will not help to stop the pandemic. As history shows, we have overcome pandemics time and time again. Along the way, we have developed new technology, made advancements in medicine and have redesigned our urban spaces and infrastructure to better cope with future pandemics. We must all do our own part in stopping a pandemic, whether it be following health guidelines or combatting misinformation. As the old saying goes, "united we stand, divided we fall". Due to the nature of infectious diseases, we are indeed all in this together.

Works Cited

Abdollahi, E., Champredon, D., Langley, J., Galvani, A., & Moghadas, S. (2020). Temporal estimates of case-fatality rate for COVID-19 outbreaks in Canada and the United States. Canadian Medical Association Journal, 192(25). doi: https://doi.org/10.1503/cmaj.200711

Ahmed, I. (2020, July 7). Hundreds of Scientists Warn COVID-19 Is Airborne, And WHO Need to Act. | Science Alert.

Ammianus Marcellinus (1940). Res Gestae (J.C. Rolfe, Trans., Vol. 2). Harvard University Press (Original work published ca. 350-400 AD).

Barberis, I., Myles, P., Ault, S. K., Bragazzi, N. L., & Martini, M. (2016). History and evolution of influenza control through vaccination: From the first monovalent vaccine to universal vaccines. Journal of Preventive Medicine and Hygiene, 57(3), E115–E120.

Barberis, I., Bragazzi, N., Galluzzo, L., & Martini, M. (2017). The history of tuberculosis: from the first historical records to the isolation of Koch's bacillus. Journal of Preventive Medicine and Hygiene, 58(1), 9-12. Retrieved from https://www.jpmh.org/index.php/jpmh

Barua, D. (1974). History of Cholera. In D. Barua & W. B. Greenough (Eds.), Cholera (1st ed., pp. 1-36). Boston, MA: Springer.

Bellhouse, D. (1998). London Plague Statistics in 1665. Journal of Official Statistics, 14(2), 207-234.

Retrieved from https://www.scb.se/contentassets/ca21efb41fee47d293bbee5bf7be7fb3/london-plague-statistics-in-1665.pdf

Benedict, C. (1988). Bubonic plague in nineteenth-century China. Modern China, 14(2), 107-155. doi: https://www.jstor.org/stable/189268

Benedictow, O. J. (2004). The Black Death, 1346-1353: The complete history. Boydell Press.

Bhalla, N. (2020, July 06). Fight climate change to prevent future pandemics like COVID-19, countries told.

Bhattacharya, S. (2005). An evaluation of current cholera treatment. Expert Opinion on Pharmacotherapy, 4(2), 141-146. doi: https://doi.org/10.1517/14656566.4.2.141

Biraben, J.-N., & LeGoff, J. (1975). The Plague in the Early Middle Ages. In R. Forster & O. Ranum (Eds.), Biology of Man in History (pp. 44-80). John Hopkins University Press.

Boak, A. E. R. (1955). Manpower Shortage and the Fall of the Roman Empire in the West. University of Michigan Press.

Boccaccio, G. Decameron (2003. G. H. McWilliam, Trans., 2nd ed.). Penguin Classics. (Original work published 1353).

Bramanti, B., Dean, K., Walloe, L., & Stenseth, N. (2019). The third plague pandemic in Europe. Proceedings of the Royal Society B: Biological Sciences, 286(1901). doi: 10.1098/rspb.2018.2429

Breman, J., & Arita, I. The confirmation and maintenance of smallpox eradication. World Health Organization. Retrieved from https://apps.who.int/iris/bitstream/handle/10665/67099/WHO_SE_80.156.pdf

Brooks, F. (1993). Revising the conquest of Mexico: smallpox, sources, and populations. The Journal of Interdisciplinary History, 24(1), 1-29. doi: 10.2307/205099

Brown, D. (2009, August 26). Lessons to be learned from 1957 pandemic. The Seattle Times.

Centers for Disease Control and Prevention. (2010, June 10). CDC Novel H1N1 Flu | The 2009 H1N1 Pandemic: Summary Highlights, April 2009-April 2010.

Centers for Disease Control and Prevention. (2016). Smallpox: Transmission. Retrieved from https://www.cdc.gov/smallpox/transmission/index.html

Centers for Disease Control and Prevention. (2018). Plague: Symptoms. Retrieved from https://www.cdc.gov/plague/symptoms/index.html

Centers for Disease Control and Prevention. (2018, March). 1918 Pandemic Influenza Historic Timeline | Pandemic Influenza (Flu) | CDC.

Centers for Disease Control and Prevention. (2019, January 22). 1957-1958 Pandemic (H2N2 virus) | Pandemic Influenza (Flu) | CDC.

Centers for Disease Control and Prevention. (2019, March 8). 2014-2016 Ebola Outbreak in West Africa | History | Ebola (Ebola Virus Disease) | CDC.

Centers for Disease Control and Prevention. (2019, May 8). 2009 H1N1 Flu Pandemic Timeline. CDC.

Centers for Disease Control and Prevention. (2019, June 11). 2009 H1N1 Pandemic. CDC

Centers for Disease Control and Prevention. (2019, December 17). The Discovery and Reconstruction of the 1918 Pandemic Virus. CDC.

Centers for Disease Control and Prevention. (2020, April). How to Protect Yourself & Others | CDC.

Centers for Disease Control and Prevention. (2020, May). Smoking and Tobacco Use | CDC.

Cummins, N., Kelly, M., & Grada, C. (2016). Living standards and plague in London, 1560-1665. Economic History Review, 69(1), 3-34. doi: https://doi.org/10.1111/ehr.12098

Cunningham, A., & Grell, O. P. (2000). The Four Horsemen of the Apocalypse: Religion, war, famine and death in Reformation Europe. Cambridge University Press.

Davies, S. (2020, May 12). This is how coronavirus could reshape our cities forever.

Defoe, D. (2009). A journal of the plague year. The Floating Press.

Dio Cassius (1927). Historiae Romanae (E. Cary, Trans., Vol. 9). Harvard University Press (Original work published ca. 180-235 AD).

Dols, M. W. (1977). The Black Death in the Middle East. Princeton University Press.

Dumbel, K., Bedson, H., & Rossier, E. (1961). Laboratory differentiation between variola major and variola minor. Bulletin of the World Health Organization, 25(1), 73-78. Retrieved from: https://www.who.int/publications/journals/bulletin/

Echenberg, M. (2011). Africa in the time of cholera: A history of pandemics from 1817 to present. (1st ed.). Cambridge, UK: Cambridge University Press.

Echenberg, M. (2002). Pestis Redux: The Initial Years of the Third Bubonic Plague Pandemic, 1894-1901. Journal of World History, 13(2), 429-449. doi: https://www.jstor.org/stable/20078978

Echenberg, M. (2010). Plague ports: The global urban impact of bubonic plague, 1894-1901 (1st ed.). New York, NY: NYU Press.

Fears, J. R. (2004). The plague under Marcus Aurelius and the decline and fall of the Roman Empire. Infectious Disease Clinics of North America 18(1), 65-77.

Gibbon, E. (1909). The Decline and Fall of the Roman Empire. Methuen and Co.

Gilliam, J. F. (1961). The Plague under Marcus Aurelius. The American Journal of Philology, 82(3), 225-251.

Halliday, S. (2001). Death and miasma in victorian London: an obstinate belief. British Medical Journal, 323(7327), 1469-1471. doi: 10.1136/bmj.323.7327.1469

Harbeck, M., Seifert, L., Hansch, S., Wagner, D. M., Birdsell, D., Parise, K. L., Wiechmann, I., Grupe, G., Thomas, A., Keim, P., Zoller, L., Bramanti, B., Riehm, J. M., & Scholz, H. C. (2013). Yersinia pestis DNA from Skeletal Remains from the 6th Century AD Reveals Insight into Justinianic Plague. PLoS Pathogens, 9(5). https://doi.org/10.1371/journal.ppat.1003349

Harper, K. (2017, December 19). How Climate Change and Plague Helped Bring Down the Roman Empire. Smithsonian Magazine. https://www.smithsonianmag.com/science-nature/how-climate-change-and-disease-helped-fall-rome-180967591/

Hays, J.N. (2005). Epidemics and Pandemics: Their impacts on human history. ABC-CLIO, Inc.

Hotez P. J. (2020). Combating antiscience: Are we preparing for the 2020s?. PLoS biology, 18(3), e3000683. https://doi.org/10.1371/journal.pbio.3000683

Ireland, N. (2020, July 28). Anti-masking groups draw from anti-vaccination playbook to spread misinformation | CBC News.

Jackson, C. (2009). History lessons: The Asian Flu pandemic. The

British Journal of General Practice, 59(565), 622–623.

Jilani, T. N., Jamil, R. T., & Siddiqui, A. H. (2020). H1N1 Influenza (Swine Flu). In StatPearls. StatPearls Publishing.

Johns Hopkins University. (2020, April). COVID-19 Map | Johns Hopkins University

Jones, D. S. (2020). History in a Crisis — Lessons for Covid-19. New England Journal of Medicine, 382(18), 1681-1683. doi:10.1056/nejmp2004361

Koplow, D. (2003). Smallpox as a biological weapon. Smallpox: The fight to eradicate a global scourge (1st ed., pp. 58-103). Berkeley, CA: University of California Press.

Kotar, S., & Gessler, J. (2013). Smallpox: A history (1st ed.) McFarland & Company, Incorporated Publishers

Ligon, B.L. (2006). Plague: A Review of its History and Potential as a Biological Weapon. Seminars in Pediatric Infectious Diseases 17(3), 161-170.

Liritzis, I. (2020). Pandemics – From Ancient Times to COVID19. Some thoughts. Mediterranean Archaeology and Archaeometry 20(1), i-ix.

Little, B. (2020, March). How the 1957 Flu Pandemic Was Stopped Early in Its Path. HISTORY.

Little, L.K. (2007). Plague and the End of Antiquity: The pandemic of 541-750. Cambridge University Press.

Littman, R.J, & Littman, M.L. (1973). Galen and the Antonine Plague. The American Journal of Philology, 94(3), 243-255.

Lu, M. C. (2020, April 17). Perspective | Future pandemics can be prevented, but that'll rely on unprecedented global cooperation.

Lubrano, A. (2020, March 24). The world has suffered through other deadly pandemics. But the response to coronavirus is unprecedented.

Mackowiak, P. A. & Sehdev, P. S. (2002). The Origin of Quarantine. Clinical Infectious Diseases 35(9): 1071-1072.

Mayo Clinic. (2019, January 10). Swine flu (H1N1 flu)—Symptoms and causes. Mayo Clinic.

Mayo Clinic. (n.d.) Tuberculosis. Retrieved from https://www.mayoclinic.org/diseases-conditions/tuberculosis/symptoms-causes/syc-20351250

McNeill, W.H. (1998). Plagues and Peoples. Anchor Books, Doubleday.

Melbourne, E. (2011). Cholera: Symptoms, Diagnosis and Treatment (1st ed.). Hauppauge, NY: Nova Science Publishers, Incorporated.

Michelakis, P. (2019). Naming the Plague in Homer, Sophocles, and Thucydides. American Journal of Philology 140(3), 381-408.

Moote, A., & Moote, D. (2006). The great plague: The story of London's most deadly year. (1st ed.). Baltimore, MD: Johns Hopkins University Press.

Morens, D. M., Daszak, P., Markel, H., & Taubenberger, J. K. (2020). Pandemic COVID-19 Joins History's Pandemic Legion. MBio, 11(3). doi:10.1128/mbio.00812-20

Mui, C. (2020, May 15). 5 Ways Our Coronavirus Recovery Strategies Might Make Or Break The Future: Part 1.

Mui, C. (2020, May 15). Making Or Breaking The Future: Part 2 - Preparing For Future Pandemics And Other Disasters (Or Not).

Newman, K. (2012). Shutt Up: Bubonic Plague and Quarantine in Early Modern England. Journal of Social History, 45(3), 809-834. Retrieved from https://www.jstor.org/stable/41678910

Niebuhr, B. G. (1849). Lectures on the History of Rome (2nd ed., Vol. III). Taylor, Walton, and Meberley.

Ochmann, S., & Roser, M. (2018). Smallpox. Retrieved from https://ourworldindata.org/smallpox

PBS. (n.d.). The First Wave | American Experience | PBS. Retrieved July 16, 2020.

Pepys, S. (1825). The diary of Samuel Pepys, complete. Retrieved from http://www.limpidsoft.com/ipad8/samuelpepys.pdf

Peters, A. (2020, March 26). How we can redesign cities to fight future pandemics.

Piot, P., & Quinn, T. C. (2013). Response to the AIDS pandemic--a global health model. The New England journal of medicine, 368(23), 2210–2218. https://doi.org/10.1056/NEJMra1201533

Pollitzer, R. (1954). Cholera studies. 1. History of the disease. Bulletin of the World Health Organization, 10(3), 421-461. Retrieved from https://www.ncbi.nlm.nih.gov/pmc/articles/PMC2542143/pdf/bullwho00557-0108.pdf

Porter, S. (2009). Plague and society. The great plague (2nd ed., pp. 7-29). Stroud, Gloucestershire: Amberly Publishing.

Porter, S. (2009). The great plague in London. The great plague (2nd ed., pp. 29-61). Stroud, Gloucestershire: Amberly Publishing.

Procopius (2005). History of the Wars (H. B. Dewing, Trans., Vol. 1). The Project Gutenburg (Original work published ca. 520-570 AD).

Pseudo-Dionysius of Tel-Mahre (1996). Chronicle, part II (W. Witakowski, Trans.). Liverpool University Press (Original work published end of 8th century AD).

Public Health Agency of Canada. (2020, June 3). Physical distancing: How to slow the spread of COVID-19 | Government of Canada.

Reuters, T. (2020, July 15). Fauci calls White House criticism of him 'bizarre' as U.S. coronavirus infections spike | CBC News.

Reuters, T. (2020, July 16). Brazil tops 2 million confirmed coronavirus cases | CBC News.

Riedel, S. (2005). Edward Jenner and the history of smallpox and vaccination. Baylor University Medical Center Proceedings, 18(1), 21-25. doi: https://doi.org/10.1080/08998280.2005.11928028

Riedel, S. (2005). Plague: from natural disease to bioterrorism. Proc Bayl University Medical Centre 18(1), 116-124.

Roos, D. (2020, March). Why the Second Wave of the 1918 Spanish Flu Was So Deadly. HISTORY.

Russell, J.C. (1968). That Earlier Plague. Demography 5(1), 174-184. doi:10.1007/bf03208570

Scott, S., & Duncan, C. J. (2004). Return of the Black Death: The world's greatest serial killer. Wiley.

Scriptores Historiae Augustae (1921. D. Magie, Trans., Vol. 1). W. Heinemann. (Original work published ca. 4th century AD).

Secon, H., Woodward, A., &; Mosher, D. (2020, June 30). A comprehensive timeline of the coronavirus pandemic at 6 months, from China's first case to the present.

Seeck, O. (1910). Geschichte des Untergangs der antiken Welt (3rd ed., Vol. I). J.B. Metzler.

Sihn, K. (2017). The 1894 plague epidemic in Hong Kong and the germ theory. Korean Journal of Medical History, 26(1), 59-94. doi: http://dx.doi.org/10.13081/kjmh.2017.26.59

Smith, G., & McFadden, G. (2002). Smallpox: Anything to declare? Nature Reviews Immunology, 2, 521-527. Retrieved from https://www.nature.com/nri/

Snowden, F. M. (2019). Epidemics and Society: From the Black Death to the present. Yale University Press.

Stathakopoulos, D. (2000). The Justinian Plague Revisited. Byzantine and Modern Greek Studies, 24(1), 256-276.

Taubenberger, J. K. (2006). The Origin and Virulence of the 1918 "Spanish" Influenza Virus. Proceedings of the American Philosophical Society, 150(1), 86–112.

Taubenberger, J. K., & Morens, D. M. (2006). 1918 Influenza: The Mother of All Pandemics. Emerging Infectious Diseases, 12(1), 15–22.

The National Archives (n.d.) The great plague 1665-1666: How did London respond to it. Retrieved from https://www.nationalarchives.gov.uk/documents/education/plague.pdf

Theves, C., Crubezy, & E., Biagini, P. (2016). History of smallpox and its spread in human populations. In M. Drancourt & D. Raoult (Eds.), Paleomicrobiology of humans (5th ed.) Washington, DC: ASM Press.

Thucydides (1881). The Peloponnesian War (B. Jowett, Trans., Vol. 1). Clarendon Press. (Original work published ca. 450-400 BC).

Tignor, R., Adelman, J., Brown, P., Elman, B., Liu, X., Pittman, H., & Shaw, B. (2014). Worlds Together, Worlds Apart, Volume 1: Beginnings to the 15th century. W.W Norton &Company.

Walsh, B. (2020, March 25). Covid-19: The history of pandemics.

Weaver, J. (2020, July 12). How the 'bureaucratic' World Health Organization ended up on the hot seat over its COVID response | CBC News.

Weekly epidemiological record. (2005). World Health Organization, 80(15), 133-140. doi: http://www.who.int/wer

Wolfe, N. (2020, April 15). How To Protect Our World From Future Pandemics.

Wolfe, R., & Sharp, L. (2002). Anti-vaccinationists past and present. British Medical Journal, 325(7361), 430-432. doi: 10.1136/bmj.325.7361.430

World Health Organization. (2017). Plague. Retrieved from https://www.who.int/news-room/fact-sheets/detail/plague

World Health Organization. (2018, July 20). Zika virus.

World Health Organization. (2019). Cholera. Retrieved from https://www.who.int/news-room/fact-sheets/detail/cholera

World Health Organization. (2020, February 10). Ebola virus disease.

World Health Organization. (2020). Tuberculosis. Retrieved from https://www.who.int/news-room/fact-sheets/detail/tuberculosis

Worsham, P.L., McGovern, T.W., Vietri, N.J., & Friedlander, A.M. (2007). Plague. In Z.F. Dembek (Ed.), Medical Aspects of Chemical and Biological Warfare (pp. 91-120). Borden Institute, Walter Reed Army Medical Center.

Zhai, P., Ding, Y., Wu, X., Long, J., Zhong, Y., & Li, Y. (2020). The epidemiology, diagnosis and treatment of COVID-19. International journal of antimicrobial agents, 55(5), 105955. https://doi.org/10.1016/j.ijantimicag.2020.105955

Zietz, B., & Dunkelberg, H. (2004). The history of the plague and the research on the causative agent Yersinia pestis. International Journal of Hygiene and Environmental Health, 207(2), 165-178. doi: https://doi.org/10.1078/1438-4639-00259

www.ingramcontent.com/pod-product-compliance
Lightning Source LLC
Chambersburg PA
CBHW030115170426
43198CB00009B/631